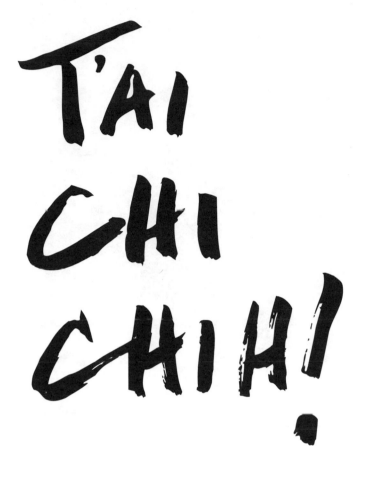

T'AI CHI CHIH!

Joy Thru Movement

By Justin F. Stone

Good Karma
Fort Yates

GOOD KARMA PUBLISHING, Inc., Publisher
P.O. Box 511
Fort Yates, ND 58538

Printed in the United States of America

First New Edition – 1996
Second Printing – Autumn 1996
Third Printing – Autumn 1997
Fourth Printing – 1999
Fifth Printing – 2000

Artwork – Ou Mie Shu
Cover calligraphy – Skip Whitson

Photography – Kimberly Grant
Back cover photo – J. Houle
Used with permission

Design and layout – Graphic Communications, Inc.
Design consulting – Dave Miranda

Library of Congress Cataloging-in-Publication Data

Stone, Justin F., 1916-
    T'ai chi chih : joy thru movement / by Justin F. Stone. -- 1st new ed.
       p.   cm.
    ISBN 1-882290-02-X (pbk.)   96-5633
    1. Ch'i kung.   I. Title.   CIP
    RA781.8.S76   1996   r96
    613.7' 148--dc20

Dedicated to my friend and teacher, Huang Wen-Shan
(philosopher, anthropologist, T'ai Chi master),
from whom I have learned so much

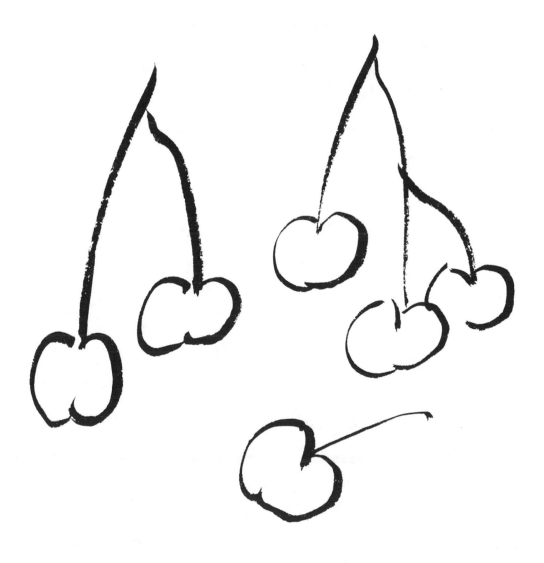

CHERRIES

The peoples of the crowded Orient generally know the feeling of "serenity in the midst of activity." It is not by refraining from action that we achieve it, but by maintaining a firm, unchanging center in the midst of disturbance.

When we do the measured movements of T'ai Chi Chih, while focusing our concentration on the spot two inches below the navel, we feel the surge of Vital Force and experience a pleasant tingling—yet, when we are quiet again, that center in the solar plexus is filled with power and we feel at rest. This serenity should spill over into our everyday lives, making possible a calm and joyous interior even during the most hectic times.

The circle represents the "Tao" or "T'ai Chi" (Supreme Ultimate)

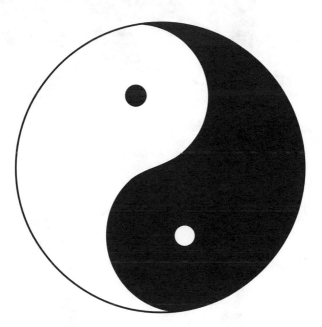

The light part is the "yang" force
(heat, expansion, the creative, masculine, positive)

The dark part is the "yin" force
(cold, contraction, the receptive, feminine, negative)

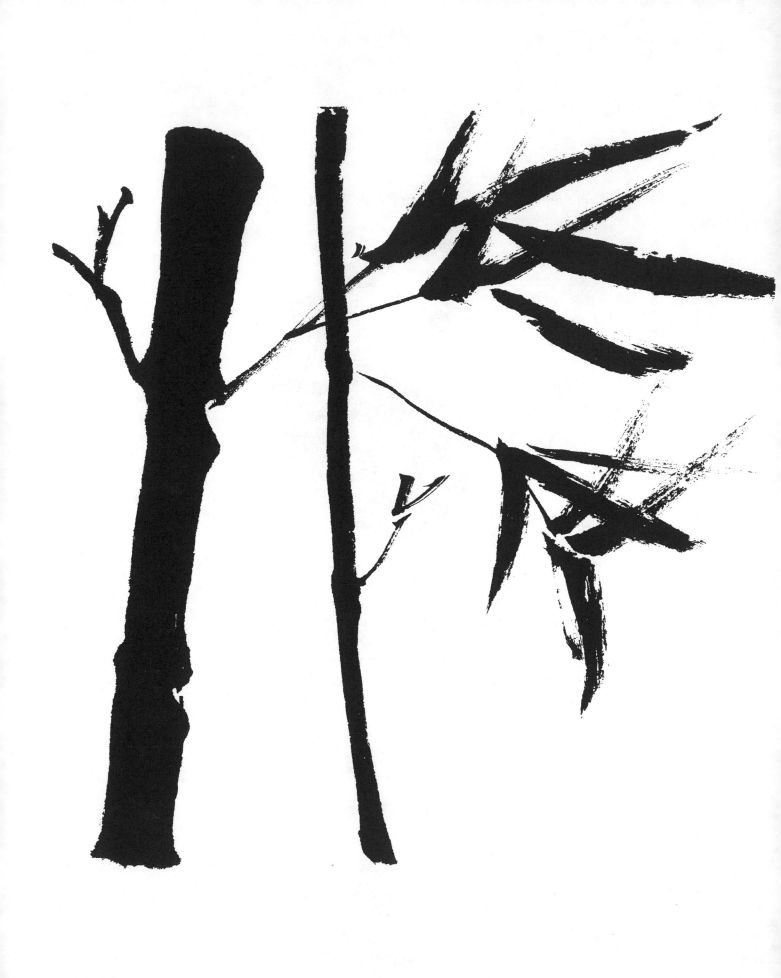

BAMBOO

Table of Contents

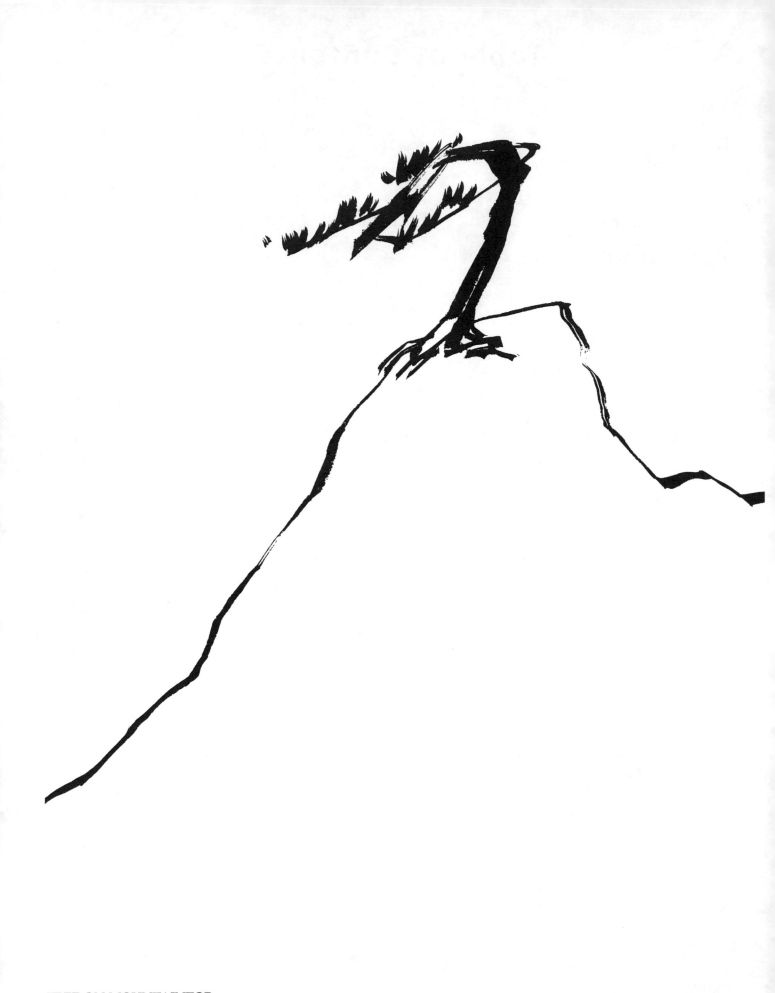

TREE ON MOUNTAINTOP

PART ONE

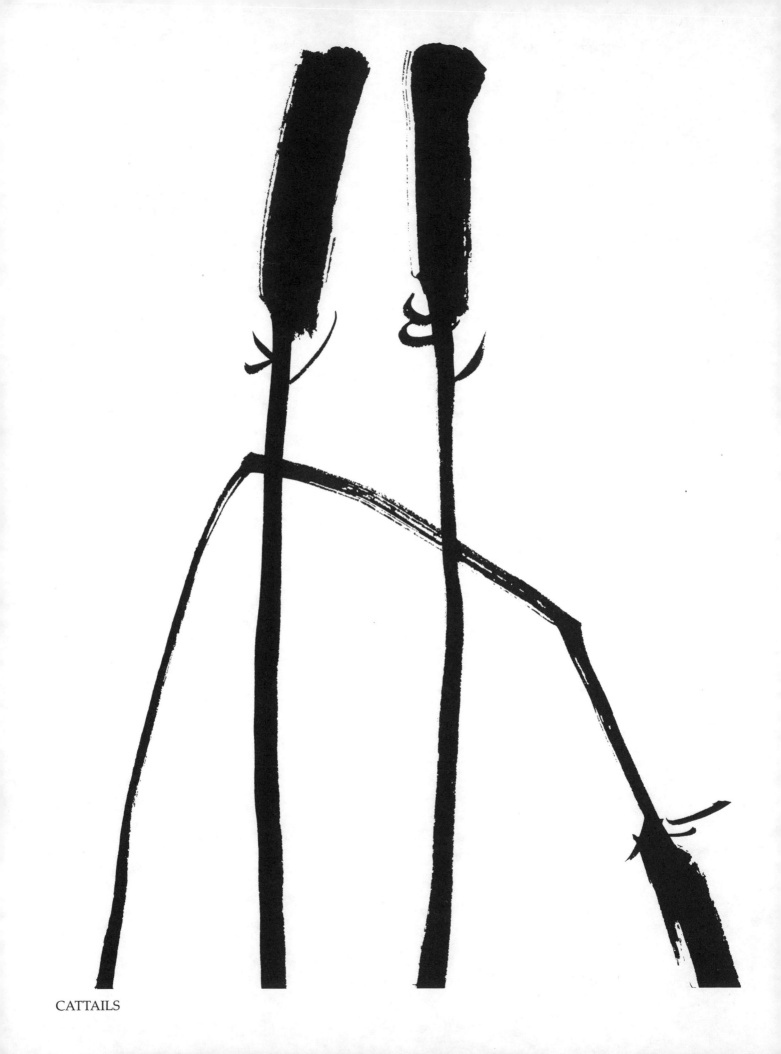

CATTAILS

Preface

What are the great secrets of life? Perhaps there are few of them. Probably none is more important than the knowledge of how to circulate and balance the Intrinsic Energy, the Vital Force of the body, known as "Chi" in Chinese. The rewards in good health, wisdom, serenity, and longevity are great for the one who learns the ancient principles and applies them in a modern way. So little of such arts is known in the West, but now, stimulated by the growth of meditation practice and the intense interest in acupuncture, people have begun to turn to ancient Chinese T'ai Chi Ch'uan, Hatha Yoga, and other forms for self-culture.

Ease of Learning T'ai Chi Chih

As a former T'ai Chi Ch'uan instructor, I am very enthusiastic about having taught this discipline, and always seemed to have a waiting list for new classes. And yet, I realize that it takes many months of hard work to learn the 108 movements of T'ai Chi Ch'uan. Once learned, it takes at least 12 feet of space in which to practise. Older people have some difficulty executing the movements, as well as a problem in memorizing the long sequence. And, finally, T'ai Chi Ch'uan, wonderful as it is, cannot be learned from a book—a personal instructor is absolutely necessary.

In contrast, T'ai Chi Chih can easily be learned from this book or my videotape. Any six of the movements, practised 36 times on the left side and 36 times on the right side, should afford great benefits. Very little space is needed; one can stand at one's desk whenever feeling drowsy and, reaching out only to arm's length, re-stimulate oneself by leisurely doing a few of the movements. They are so gentle, and take so little coordination, that people of any age can easily do them. All that is needed is to practise the movements regularly, 10 or 15 minutes in the morning and 10 or 15 minutes in the late afternoon or early evening. Properly done, the result should be a flow of energy and a feeling of well-being somewhat like the aftermath of an internal bath. The first manifestation is usually a tingling in the fingers and a feeling of fullness and energy-flow in the hands. If the mental concentration is kept in the soles of the feet (the so-called "Bubbling Spring") or two inches below the navel (the "T'an T'ien," pronounced "Dantienne"), the flow will eventually surge through the body, and a feeling of heat may suddenly appear in the arms, at the base of the skull, or elsewhere. A vibration may begin in the soles of the feet, or at the solar plexus, and there may be a feeling that the hairs at the top of the neck are standing up. A strong twitching is often felt in the forehead just above and between the eyes, a spot usually referred to in occult circles as "the Third Eye." Each person will feel the surge of Vital Force in his or her own way, and it is a pleasant feeling. This heat current is also said to be very healing in nature, and I can attest to such effects in my own particular case as regards a chronic ailment, probably resulting from injury. Above all, we tend to "wake up," to feel good and more alive. In this respect, T'ai Chi Chih is like a valuable meditation.

What is Chi?

What is this Vital Force that we become aware of, the flow of Intrinsic Energy seeming to arise within us? The Chinese, those people of great vitality, call it Chi. It is known as Ki in Japan, where it is the basis for higher Aikido and other martial arts. The wise men of India have referred to it variously as Sakti, Kundalini, and Prana. In Indian Tantric practices, this energy as Sakti (the active force of the reality, Shiva) is actually worshiped. Taking this energy up along the spine, opening the psychic centers, is the way for humans to become gods, in the Kundalini practice of Hindu Tantra, but this must be done under close supervision of a Perfect Master (Guru), so its possibilities are limited to only a few.

It is interesting that the Chinese use the word Chi as translation for the Indian Sanskrit Prana, all the force of the universe, the power that breathes us and makes us live. (This same force is expressed, unfortunately, in the atom bomb.) This Chi is also used as translation for the Sanskrit word Prajna, which means wisdom in the greater sense. So the Vital Force, this Intrinsic Energy, is also the wisdom that is the deep-rooted source of intuition. A long-time practicer of T'ai Chi Chih will know well what the ancients meant when they said, "To unite the Divine Energy within me with the Universal Energy, that is the Goal!"

Power of Chi Circulation

Hakuin Zenji, the 18th century Japanese Zen Master (and perhaps the most influential in Japan's long history of Buddhism), tells a curious story in his little-known work, *The Yasenkanna*. Tired and in extremely bad health from his arduous meditations and long search for truth, Hakuin heard about a Sennin, a mountain Master, living in seclusion near Shirokawa (White River Junction) in the mountains of Japan. He promptly made a pilgrimage there and, after difficulty in finding the Master (who was living in a cave in the remote recesses of the mountains), he finally came face-to-face with him in his small retreat. Hakuin was surprised to see no food at all in the cave, and he knew, from the villagers, that Hakuyu, the Master, had not left there for some time. Moreover, the older man (some said he had been the teacher of another great Master over 100 years before!) was wearing but a thin covering, curled with cold (I can attest to the freezing winter weather in those mountains!) and yet did not seem to notice the chill at all. He was kneeling in meditation when Hakuin entered the cave, practising the Naikan discipline (explained as Nei Kung, the Chinese pronunciation, in my book *Meditation for Healing*) that is part of the Chi Kung series of

practices, just as T'ai Chi Chih is. These practices are designed to activate, circulate, and balance the Divine Energy (Chi) lying dormant in each one of us.

Hakuyu taught this circulation of the Chi to Hakuin, both to help his rapidly-degenerating health and to enable him to make a break-through in his contemplations, necessary for him to reach full Enlightenment. Hakuin writes that, using this method of circulating and balancing the Chi, he succeeded in both endeavors and went on to become one of the greatest Zen Masters the Orient has known. Since Hakuin was one of the most notable religious figures in Japanese history, and since he was of a people well-known for their understatement, can we doubt his word when he attests to the efficacy of the flowing Chi?

Balancing Yin and Yang

When we speak of "balancing" this Intrinsic Energy (which Chinese Zennists sometimes obscurely referred to as "your original face"), we mean bringing the yin and yang elements into balance. In Chinese cosmology, we have the ineffable "Tao" (also known as "T'ai Chi"), the Supreme Ultimate about which nothing can be predicated. From this matrix come the yin and the yang, which can be called the negative and the positive, the receptive and the creative, the cold and the hot, the insubstantial and the substantial, the feminine and the masculine, etc.—the forces of the two polarities. Then, from the yin and yang we get heaven above, earth below, and humankind in the center. (This is why Japanese flower arrangements are generally three-pointed.) From these derive the 10,000 things, the world of diversified phenomena perceived by the senses.

The ancient teaching is that the yin (feminine) and yang (masculine) elements separate when in motion, and come together again in qui-escence. So, when we begin the motions of T'ai Chi Chih, we are dividing the two forces; then we balance them as we practise. Finally, when we are still again, they reunite.

Often we see the great teaching represented by the ball that appears like this:

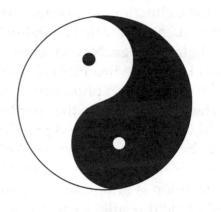

This is the Tao, or T'ai Chi. Notice that in the dark (the feminine or negative) there is a faint spot of light, and, conversely, in the light (the masculine or positive), there is a faint spot of dark.Thus there is always some feminine in the masculine, and vice versa. It is this which makes possible the balancing of the Chi.

The Chinese say that when one force is carried to extremes (grows too strong), it turns into its opposite. This is possible because yin and yang attract each other. So, too much yang (positive) eventually becomes yin (negative). We can easily identify this in our own world, where it is said, "Pleasure indefinitely prolonged becomes pain." One ice cream soda tastes good, but ten ice cream sodas make us sick. And so it is said that, "The wise person goes to his or her triumph like a funeral," knowing the greatest high eventually turns into a low. The Sage has said, "If you want to lift anything, first push down on it to break the attachment." The yang (creative) is the father of all things, but the yin (receptive) is the great mother. Each eventually turns into its opposite, and both are always present to some degree.

Water, and most fluids, is strongly yin, and when we have an excess of fluid in our systems, we are too yin and tend toward illness. The flow of the Chi in T'ai Chi Chih helps dry this excess fluid, so we tend to lose weight if we are overweight and to have better health as this extra yin is removed. We are usually thirsty after practising T'ai Chi Chih because of this drying effect. It is best not to drink something cold immediately after finishing, as we have been exercising the internal organs and producing a subtle heat in them.

Effective Use of Balanced Energy

When we first start the movements of T'ai Chi Chih, we are beginning to circulate the Chi. As we emphasize right or left in the hands, to balance the substantial or insubstantial position of the legs (through the knees), we are balancing this Vital Force as it flows. Then, when we come to rest, the yin and yang elements reunite and are stored in the bones, according to the old Chinese teaching. It is this stored Chi energy that enables a Master of Karate, Aikido, or the other martial art disciplines, to smash a hand through a concrete block, a stunt witnessed many times by Westerners. (Not too long ago a building was destroyed in Japan in this manner, using only the hands of a few adepts who volunteered their services.) It is not muscular force the adept uses; you will note the person usually lets out a sharp cry as he or she musters the stored Chi and then smashes the hand through the obstacle. Concentrating on the T'an T'ien (two inches below the navel) will cause a good deal of Chi to be stored there, the seat of heaven. There are Aikido clubs in Japan whose members go swimming on the coldest winter days, keeping intensive concentration on the heat-making Chi stored in the spot below the navel ("Tanden" in Japanese).

Shall I relate one more story to show the wondrous properties of the Chi? It is a story that was told to me (I was not there), but one that is fairly common in circles of this Oriental discipline. Two black belt Judo adepts heard that an older Master was coming to a city close to theirs. They made a hurried trip there to pay their respects, and were somewhat disappointed to find a tiny, older man, perhaps weighing less than 100 pounds. The first Judo man, over six feet tall and quite muscular, said to the Master, "All my life I have been hearing about the power of this Chi. Would you be kind enough to demonstrate the power to us?"

The Master thought for a moment. "I'll tell you what," he began, "You two come at me from different directions and throw me down!"

The two big men, much younger than the little fellow, were astonished. "We'll kill you!" exclaimed one of them.

"And do me the honor of not taking it easy with me!" continued the Master.

The two Judo men huddled to discuss the turn of events. "You flip him and I'll catch him before he hits the mat," suggested one, and the other nodded. "We don't want to hurt the little fellow."

The two separated, turned, and began to advance on the Master, watching his breathing and waiting for the right time to spring. When they did move, it was quickly—and then, I am told, the spectators saw a strange sight. One man was immediately seen lying on the ground ten feet away, his glasses knocked off, "looking for the freight train," as he put it. The other had staggered back against the wall, and a small fleck of blood appeared at his nostrils. What is most surprising is that none of the assembled spectators had seen the little man move at all!

This, of course, is an extreme example of the effective use of the Vital Force. And yet, it is latent in all of us. The storing of this force below the navel is what enables the Holy Man, in Tibet or northern India, to walk through the snow and ice on the coldest days, comfortable wearing nothing but a loincloth. It is known as the "Dumo heat" in Tibetan Tantric Buddhism. And it is the force used by healers, who may impart it as a healing energy (felt as heat) by a technique of laying-on-of-hands, or something similar (as in the very effective Johrei of the Japanese Healing Church, Sekai Kyusei Kyo). This same energy that seems to heal is the basis of all sexual vigor, which is said to be greatly enhanced by the practice of T'ai Chi Chih.

So, circulation and balance of the Chi energy is one of the great secrets of life, open to any of us who will make the effort. Most do not have the time (or inclination) to practise extreme disciplines, such as Tantric Kundalini Yoga or Advanced Hatha Yoga. Nevertheless, we can balance and circulate this Intrinsic Life Force (which the great Indian philosopher, Shankara, called "The Real") through the simple practice of T'ai Chi Chih. If the student practises faithfully, the results can be great. Without making much effort, we cannot hope to achieve much. Repetition is important. Regular practice is needed to yield results—and it is well worth the effort! So, in this way, we can utilize one of the great secrets of life.

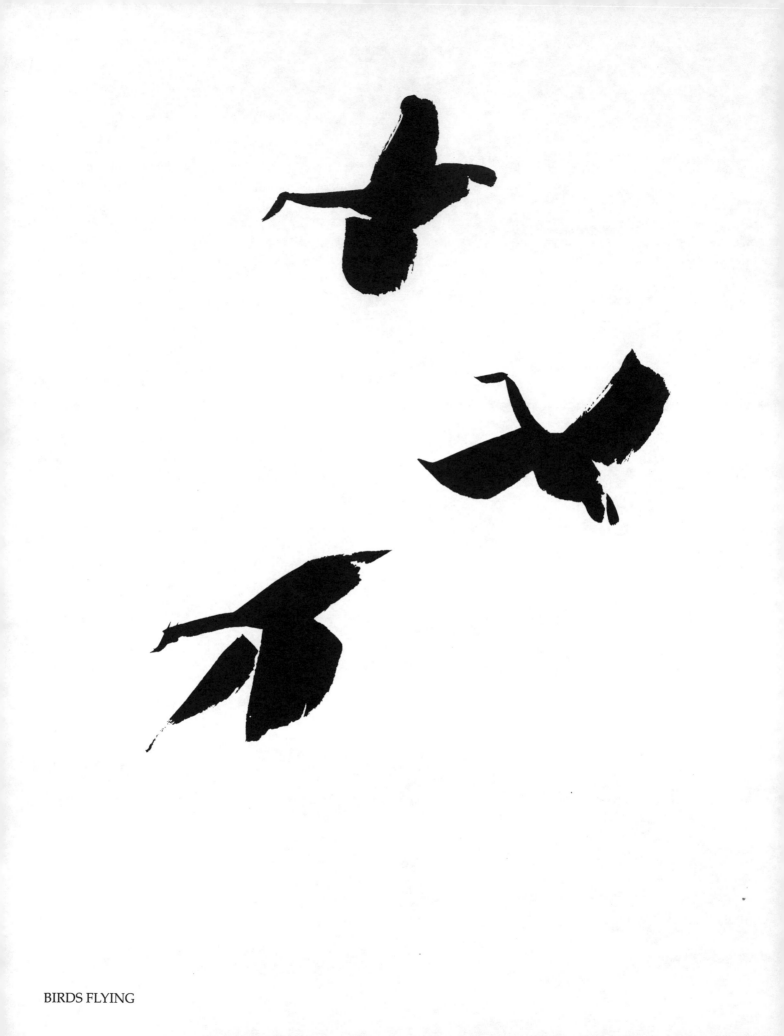

BIRDS FLYING

Foreword

We are very logical and intellectual in the West. But when we try to fit T'ai Chi Chih into a neat definition, or hold on to our own personal ideas about it, we miss its essence. Trying to categorize it is like three blind men describing an elephant while each holds on to a different part of it. T'ai Chi Chih is at once personal and impersonal, physical and ethereal. It is not an exercise, and yet it is the best "exercise" you can do. (Unlike exercise, though, it will not tire you.)

T'ai Chi Chih consists of 19 gentle, graceful movements and one pose that can be done by almost anyone. Working with the building blocks of the universe—yin and yang, which when combined become the Tao, the essence of all life—Justin created this new form of movement. The results we experience by doing the movements speak of Justin's conscious intention to end pain and suffering. This is a tall order. Yet without that focus we spend our lives disgruntled, feeling that something is missing. What is important about our lives? What meaning is there to our being here?

We have a tendency to separate our mind, body, and emotions. But the true demonstration of spiritual growth is integrating these three elements and then bringing them to bear in a situation. How do we develop a foundation for this integration and wholeness? The key is T'ai Chi Chih. Through T'ai Chi Chih we gain the balance that allows us to see clearly and to act with integrity. Up until this time we have seen "through a glass, darkly." Clarity allows us to experience the essential beauty of life.

The effects of T'ai Chi Chih are cumulative. Therefore, consistency of practice is vital in order to experience the maximum benefits. And yet, many students quickly experience peace and clarity. I have observed during my many years as an accredited teacher that although students come to T'ai Chi Chih class tired and stressed, they leave with renewed physical and mental energy. Specific benefits vary with each person, but the benefits are usually precisely what each individual needs.

Justin F. Stone is a gentleman and a gentle man. He generously shares his deep understanding and life experiences. Such understanding is usually gleaned only after many years of following the path of a monk or yogi. Justin is a modern Renaissance man and citizen of the world. A former financial analyst, big band leader, and composer, he has also been a seeker in Japan, and a holy man in India. Now 80 years old, Justin is a prolific painter and jazz composer. He maintains an active schedule lecturing and conducting T'ai Chi Chih seminars and workshops around the country. He opens the way to wisdom with skill, grace, and joy. To do T'ai Chi Chih with Justin is to know that life reveals itself joyously. His continual presence in my life has been a source of inspiration and love.

In this newly revised textbook, we are introduced to the wonder of T'ai Chi Chih. The author, photographer, and publisher have put together an invaluable collection of stop-action photographs with simple instruction. The book, however, is only an aid. To experience T'ai Chi Chih you must do it. As it is said in the Orient, and as Justin is fond of saying, "You can't appease the hunger by reading the menu." Through T'ai Chi Chih the great adventure unfolds daily as we do our practice and discover answers to questions that have long been held, gently in trust, deep within our being. Let the journey begin.

Carmen L. Brocklehurst
Albuquerque, New Mexico
April 1997

Publisher's note: Carmen Brocklehurst hosts the public television series on T'ai Chi Chih, which continues to air in many U.S. localities.

New Introduction

Having practised* the ancient T'ai Chi Ch'uan for many years and having taught it at universities and elsewhere, I finally realized that the form is difficult for most people to learn and almost impossible for some people to do. The benefits are many and the satisfactions great *if* one spends the long time necessary to master it and begin to realize the effects of circulating and balancing the Chi, the Intrinsic Energy sometimes referred to as Vital Force. I found, through conversations with other T'ai Chi Ch'uan instructors, that for every 15 people who begin T'ai Chi Ch'uan lessons, perhaps one will be motivated enough to learn the first two sections, and often none go on to master the three divisions of 108 movements in the Yang system. So, although I recognized the benefits of practising T'ai Chi Ch'uan and received these benefits daily, it was all too apparent that great numbers of people would not do T'ai Chi Ch'uan, that it was for a comparative few in this country.

Believing strongly in the benefits of the ancient yin-yang system and having observed in myself the considerable gains from circulation and balancing of the Chi, I began, around 1969, to experiment with my own forms based on the ancient principles, forms that did not have to be performed in any order and yet would bring great benefits, even if only some of them were learned and practised. Having been fortunate enough to learn several little-known movements from an old Chinese man—movements practised in former days—I used these as the starting point for my experiments. One, later known as "Circles within Circles," I dropped as it seemed too difficult for the average person to successfully perform. I changed the other two movements and added my own leg movements, with the "yinning" and "yanging" now so familiar to the thousands of those who practise my form, T'ai Chi Chih. These two, along with the swinging movement known as "Rocking Motion," I taught to my T'ai Chi Ch'uan students to do as preliminary warm-up "exercises" before beginning T'ai Chi Ch'uan. The students seemed much

taken with the new movements, and there was considerable enthusiasm for them.

Over the next few years, a time when I personally was doing considerable meditation and other spiritual practice, new movements came to me in an effortless manner. I tried to name them in simple, descriptive terms. When enough had been perfected, I decided to call them, collectively, "T'ai Chi Chih," T'ai Chi being generally translated as "Supreme Ultimate" (same as "Tao") and the character for Chih meaning "knowledge" or "knowing." (Chinese has no grammar and the same word can be a verb, a noun, or an adjective.) So we were now dealing with "Knowledge of the Supreme Ultimate," and an apt description it is. My studies in India, Japan and Chinese cities had led me to believe that control of the Chi (known as "Prana" in India) was the great secret of life. Indeed, the Indian Sage, Sri Aurobindo, had made the audacious statement that if the universe were abolished, this Chi would be capable of constructing a new universe in its place! Elsewhere in this book and in some of my other books, I comment in great detail about the Chi and what it really is and does.

In 1974, Sun Publishing Company asked me to write a book on T'ai Chi Ch'uan, my first two books (*The Joys of Meditation* and *Abandon Hope*) having been unexpectedly successful for them. I declined and countered with the suggestion that I do a book, the first, on T'ai Chi Chih. This suggestion was enthusiastically accepted, and I began the laborious task of finishing and naming the 19 forms which appeared in the first T'ai Chi Chih book. (Later "Bird Flaps its Wings" was added, making 20 in all.) When this task was completed, I began to write the book, which featured a foreword by the great Chinese scholar, Huang Wen-Shan. I worked with Sun Publishing to produce the necessary photographs. The task was completed and the book published a few months before the first formal lessons in T'ai Chi Chih were given in Albuquerque, New Mexico.

Naturally, T'ai Chi Chih teaching methods have evolved as classes proliferated, and the order in which the movements were taught gradually changed until they have stabilized in the sequence

Editor's note: The author uses "practise" as a verb and "practice" as a noun.

given in this new edition, complete with all new photographs and instruction.

In August 1975, T'ai Chi Chih Teachers' Training classes began and have continued ever since at an average of three or four a year. Here eager aspirants who had mastered T'ai Chi Chih forms and who were receiving the benefits from their own practice, attended concentrated courses designed to show them how to teach T'ai Chi Chih and were constructed so as to give them background knowledge of the philosophy on which T'ai Chi Chih is based. As of mid-1996, about 1,100 instructors have been accredited after successfully completing the necessary training. They, in turn, went to work with students in their own classes as they fanned out across the United States and through some foreign countries, such as Switzerland, West Germany, Chile and Canada. Much has been learned from *their* experiences in teaching, and I am grateful to them for advancing our knowledge of this new form, now only 22 years old.

When it became apparent that the order in which T'ai Chi Chih movements are taught in class was somewhat different from the way they appeared in the original book, it was obvious that a revised edition would have to be compiled to bring in the new movements ("Bird Flaps its Wings" and the "Six Healing Sounds") and to adjust the order of movements in the book to that which now predominates in class teaching. These new developments had evolved from actual teaching experiences, and it is necessary that T'ai Chi Chih, like all growing forms, evolve and not remain stagnant. To remain unchanging is to die.

This book has been written to fill that need. As mentioned, the movements performed with the "Six Healing Sounds" have changed slightly, and "Bird Flaps its Wings" was added to the original 19 movements. The overly difficult "Circles within Circles," which is not taught in classes, has been removed from this new edition. T'ai Chi Chih is justifiably called "Joy thru Movement," and we want it to be fun; there is no need to force difficult forms on the beginning student. Actually the practice of any ten of the 20 movements and postures, if repeated regularly, should be enough

to bring great results, but, of course, it is more advantageous to learn *all* the movements and get the benefits from each. It is felt that this book now faithfully coincides with the T'ai Chi Chih that is taught by teachers in classes, and whether the reader learns alone, from this book or my videotape, or studies in T'ai Chi Chih classes, he or she should find the book to be a faithful text, particularly with the addition of the many photographs which clearly indicate the sequence of each movement.

This is the background on how T'ai Chi Chih came into being and why this new book was written. These are not ancient forms; they were originated by me, but they do use the very old yin-yang principles and a few ideas from T'ai Chi Ch'uan. The purpose was, and is, to provide easily learned movements that afford the practicer great benefits. How great these benefits are—spiritually, physically and psychologically—we did not know at the beginning, and it has been gratifying through the years to constantly receive new reports of hitherto unsuspected benefits experienced by those learning T'ai Chi Chih.

Whether one understands the reasons for such benefits or not and whether or not one has faith, regular practice of T'ai Chi Chih should bring great rewards. Just do it and let your own experience convince you. Many have stated that they like T'ai Chi Chih because no beliefs are needed and words play no part in successful practice. Truly, the aim is "Joy thru Movement," and such movement is easy. Moreover, the complete form can easily be learned in the eight or ten lessons usually constituting a complete beginner's course, which takes merely a matter of a few weeks to complete. T'ai Chi Chih can be a loving, as well as a healing, experience. Teachers' training aspirants do not soon forget the great feeling of warmth that grows between themselves and their instructors, and most seem to leave the teachers' courses on a real high, which, hopefully, they pass along to their students. We trust the reader of this book will join us in this simple practice. If enough people do T'ai Chi Chih, we might even have peace and love in the world.

PART TWO

General Instruction

The movements, and their variations, that you are about to learn are the results of many years of experimentation. From a development of the original two movements shown me, adding the leg motions and making other changes, I expanded and added 18 more, giving them descriptive names wherever possible. I have chosen practical, rather than poetic, names for the different movements. When we speak of "Around the Platter," it is not difficult to envision the hands moving in a circular manner. Likewise, "Push Pull" is very graphic, if not particularly elegant. The purpose of the names is to clearly identify the movements and help you remember them.

Drawing on my meditation experiences and T'ai Chi Ch'uan training, I intuitively devised the other movements, some of which vaguely resemble parts of T'ai Chi Ch'uan. This is not surprising, as both are Chi Kung disciplines, based on the great yin-yang principles.

Studying with a Teacher

Many have learned T'ai Chi Chih from the book or videotape alone, but it is helpful to have instruction by a fully accredited (certified) teacher. Those who are accredited studied—and subsequently practised—the 20 movements on a regular basis for some time, then took the intensive Teachers' Training class. Not all those who took such a class were certified, however. If the reader is to study with a teacher (in a group or singly), it is best to be sure the teacher is an accredited one. Self-proclaimed teachers do not have the experience or the understanding of the complex principles involved, and nobody has approved their own personal practice in the traditional Oriental manner.

Healing Resulting from T'ai Chi Chih

Since the first lessons in T'ai Chi Chih were given in 1974, there have been many reports of wondrous healings and gratifying spiritual experiences. An exceptional woman in northern California suffered from bone cancer of the leg, and had to take her first lessons in T'ai Chi Chih while seated. By the end of her eight-lesson course, taken with a very good certified teacher, she was standing and doing the leg movements. Subsequent strict and regular practice brought great improvement in her condition and she had the courage to go on and take the intensive Teachers' Training course. Today she is an effective, accredited teacher, with many changes in her life. She is not the only one to have had such an experience, though the real benefits of T'ai Chi Chih go far beyond such physical welfare. People with high blood pressure, weight problems, sexual difficulties, and many other chronic ailments report quick and marked improvement. The secret is to do the movements correctly and to practise regularly.

Body Posture for Successful Practice

We are relaxed and the hands are soft. The air is felt to be very heavy as the hands move through it, fingers spread apart. This may appear contradictory, but it is not. It is easy to feel the air as heavy and still keep the hands slightly cupped and relaxed.

The air being very heavy, we have the feeling of "swimming" through the dense atmosphere as we move in slow, leisurely fashion from beginning to end of each movement. Usually we repeat each movement 9, 18 or 36 times on each side.

This feeling of swimming through very heavy air, with the resultant surge of energy and tingling in the fingers, will eventually bring us the firm conviction that this seemingly "empty" universe is actually a vast continuum of intelligence and energy. When we realize this, we have reached a high stage of development. At such time the energy appears to be flowing and we are just shaping it.

In the beginning we are apt to focus too much on the hands, while, in truth, it is the legs which are "yinning" and "yanging." It is vital that we bend the knees and shift our weight from the left to right and back again. Unlike T'ai Chi Ch'uan, in many movements of T'ai Chi Chih the back heel comes off the ground as we go forward and the front toe lifts off the ground as the weight settles back. At all times the torso, from the waist up, is held straight, though not rigid, no matter how much the knees bend (almost like a fencer's pose, it might seem) and no matter how much the waist turns on those movements which call for a waist turn. Important! The head and torso are held in an erect position in most movements, with the head as though suspended from the ceiling by wires.

In T'ai Chi Chih, most movements are circular. Sometimes there are subtle circles within circles, as, when we push forward, we dip our arms slightly and then bring them up again, making an imperceptible circular movement down to the floor. This circularity is one of the secrets of the energy generated, and is part of the "continuity" I so often speak of. When we push forward (as in the movement called "Push Pull"), we dip the hands slightly so there is a gentle arc ⌣. Thus we make small circles, and sometimes there are circles within circles.

Most beginners do not use the wrists and hands enough, preferring to make cumbersome arm movements. Actually, most of the T'ai Chi Chih movements are performed with the wrists, which are kept loose and pliable. Fingers are slightly spread apart, the hands slightly cupped as though around the sides of a ball, and there is complete relaxation from the waist up. Conversely, the foot that is flat on the floor is firm, as though gripping the ground with the sole of the foot.

Preliminary Movements

The first two movements are called "Rocking Motion" and "Bird Flaps its Wings." The gently undulating "Rocking Motion" is vaguely derived from a practice that older people in Taiwan and China have frequently performed, sometimes as much as 2,000 times a day. It is an excellent preliminary movement as it really starts the circulation going. The original movement the older people did was somewhat more restricted and has been called the "Dharma tendon-building" motion, probably pointing to a Buddhist origin. I remember one time recommending that a man who had suffered a stroke do nothing but "Rocking Motion" as I have evolved it, without worrying about trying to execute the other movements in this book. He was told to do it 1,000 times a day and found it to be very beneficial.

The movement itself is relaxing and refreshing. And if one remembers that the air is "very heavy" as the arms swing forward (palms up), and then swing back again (palms down), he or she should begin to feel a tingling in the fingers as the Chi begins to circulate.

"Bird Flaps its Wings" was a latecomer, not appearing in the original edition of the book. I originated it after the first T'ai Chi Chih lessons had been given in 1974, and subsequent practice found it to be a very beneficial movement, with slightly different effects than appear in other motions. This is not surprising as each set of movements seems to have a slightly different effect, adding up to a complete and well-rounded whole as all, or most, of the movements are mastered and practised regularly.

"Rocking Motion" should be performed effortlessly for two or three minutes before going on to "Bird Flaps its Wings." No need to count the number of times. With "Bird Flaps its Wings," each group of three, with the wrists revolving and the hands spinning forward and around once on the third time, makes one complete set. This set of three can be repeated three or six times—or more if desired—as part of the morning routine. One can think of "Rocking Motion" and "Bird Flaps its Wings" as "preliminary" or warm-up movements before going on to the main body of movements that begins with "Around the Platter."

Leg Motions

In the following moves, there are basically two leg motions. First we have the forward and back motion, on the left and on the right, with the right heel coming off the ground and then the left toe—vice versa on the right side. The sideways step, where we slightly bend the knee, step to the side, and come down on the heel and then the sole of the foot, we call the "T'ai Chi Step." Most, but not all, of the main body of movements use one or the other of these leg movements, and the "yinning" and "yanging" of the legs as we shift the weight to "substantial" and "insubstantial" (yang and yin) is extremely important. It is the legs that shift the weight.

Don't try to do T'ai Chi Chih stiff-legged! There should be a gentle rocking motion in the forward-and-back leg motions. The motions are easy and natural. In the sideways "T'ai Chi Step," used in such movements as "Carry the Ball to the Side" and "Pulling Taffy," the heel must touch the ground before the foot flattens. Do not just fall sideways, but lift the leg slightly, bend the knee, and bring the heel down first.

Practice Program

Unlike T'ai Chi Ch'uan, where we have to learn and master all movements and memorize the entire 16-18 minute sequence of 108 movements (some are repetitions), in T'ai Chi Chih we only have to learn five or six of the movements in this book and do them regularly (perhaps twenty minutes in the morning and ten minutes later in the day), 18 times on both left and right sides, to gain the benefit. So there is not much to learn. It is application—constant daily practice—that gets results.

The practicer may choose whatever movements appeal to him or her and seem to circulate the most Chi. (Note the tingling in the fingers and hands.) A typical program, beginning with the "Rocking Motion" and "Bird Flaps its Wings," would go on to encompass "Around the Platter" (perhaps 18 times on each side), "Bass Drum" (also 18 times), "Daughter on the Mountaintop" and "Daughter in the Valley" (18 times), and two of the variations of "Pulling Taffy" (three times each). You might close with "Passing Clouds" (nine times) and the "Six Healing Sounds," followed by the stationary "Cosmic Consciousness Pose," held three to five minutes.

The reader will probably want to make his or her own program. Try to do at least 25-30 minutes a day, with particular emphasis on doing T'ai Chi Chih immediately upon arising. Once you get in the habit of beginning the day this way, you will almost surely miss it if you have to skip one day. And notice the salutary effect such practice has on the regularity of the bowels. T'ai Chi Chih is one of the few ways to exercise the internal organs.

If there is sufficient time, it is, of course, beneficial to do all 20 of the movements. There is no particular effort involved in the movements, so fatigue should not be a factor. Actually, it seems as if one has more energy at the finish of the practice period than he or she had at the beginning.

T'ai Chi Chih motions can be performed at any speed. Generally speaking, slow, gentle movements will stir up and circulate the most Chi, and the leisurely pace will enable the practicer to bend his or her knees and shift the weight without difficulty. However, one should experiment with different speeds and choose whatever seems most effective personally.

Function and Essence

Standing in the "Cosmic Consciousness Pose" for a while after finishing the movements will bring one to a period of rest in which the yin and yang Chi, which separated while the practicer was in motion, have a chance to flow together again and become integrated and balanced.

The Chinese speak of "function" when the Intrinsic Energy is in motion, the yin and yang separating. They also speak of "essence" when the yin and yang flow together again and there is an inner stillness. For full integration of mind and body, it is best to practise both function and essence, or movement followed by stillness. The "Cosmic Consciousness Pose" will help effect this balance, and the meditation instruction ("Great Circle Meditation") on pp. 94-95 can also help one achieve reintegration after the movements are stilled. These are important secrets, and it is up to the reader to avail him or herself of them as one wishes.

Additional Tips

My T'ai Chi Ch'uan master used to say, "Try to have no extraneous thoughts while practising." In other words, put your concentration in the soles of the feet or below the navel (whichever is easier), and, if possible, keep it there. Empty the mind before beginning; forget troubles and other preoccupation. The great Chinese philosopher, Chuang Tzu, spoke of the "fasting mind." We keep our heads too cluttered and accumulate too much tension; let the mind fast a bit for 15 minutes!

After we have practised T'ai Chi Chih for some time, we can increase the flow of our Vital Force by visualizing all the energy of the universe coming in through our extended fingers as we move. The Tibetans—and northern Indians—say there are five colored Pranas (energies), and seeing these flow individually into the tips of the fingers will heighten the electric feeling, but this should not be attempted in the beginning. After practising T'ai Chi Chih for some years, the student may notice a slight trembling in the fingers as he or she performs the movements. Certainly the practicer is not nervous! This is a favorable sign that the Intrinsic Energy is flowing smoothly through the meridian channels, and it means that the practicer has reached an advanced stage of development.

Give yourself to T'ai Chi Chih for 30 minutes each day. Practise regularly. The Chinese say, "You cannot appease the hunger by reading the menu!" It is only through practice that you get rich rewards. It is my feeling that the circulation of the Chi is one of life's great secrets. So, master the simple movements and practise them regularly. Good luck!

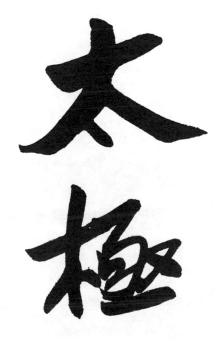

Important Points on Moving Correctly

For the beginning student the most important aspect is to learn *how* to move. It is of utmost importance that T'ai Chi Chih be practised correctly in accordance with the principles of yin-yang so that results will be maximized. Knowing where to place the arms and feet will come easily, but eager students often try too hard and use considerable effort, causing tension when T'ai Chi Chih must be tension-free. Any tension will keep the Chi (Intrinsic Energy) from flowing freely through the meridian channels.

The student must not think of T'ai Chi Chih as "exercise." In truth it is the best exercise I know, since it exercises the internal organs and does not tire one but tends to increase energy. However, it is all-important that T'ai Chi Chih be done *softly*, without effort—what we call "the effort of no effort."

If you will remember to think of yourself as moving slow motion in a dream or slowly swimming through heavy air, yet without exertion, you will have the idea of how to move.

The movements are not done rhythmically like a dance. Long, sweeping, "graceful" movements are apt to be all yin or all yang, thus negating the practice. Rather, the motions are performed almost leisurely as though the relaxed student is more of an onlooker than a participant.

The correct posture is that of standing with the tailbone pressed slightly forward, and the T'an T'ien (two inches below the navel) compressed against the backbone. The shoulders are relaxed and drooping, and the hands and wrists (more than the arms) move in soft, circular motions. "Softness and continuity" are necessary. Nice and even, like the chewing of food, is one description the ancient teachers used. Breathing is natural.

The practicer must keep his or her concentration in the soles of the feet (easy) or on the spot two inches below the navel (more difficult) while doing the movements. The "Heart Fire" (the Great Yang of the heart, corresponding to the yang of the sun) should be brought down; otherwise the Yin of the kidneys (corresponding to the yin of the moon) will rise. It is not desirable to have the water section floating upward. The great benefits in health, increased energy and serenity come from bringing the Heart Fire down as the Chi circulates. When the reader becomes familiar with the practice, these points will become clear.

There are three confirming signs in learning and practising T'ai Chi Chih: first, the practicer will note that his or her fingers begin to tremble a bit while moving; perhaps friends may call attention to this. It means the Intrinsic Energy is now flowing freely.

Secondly, after some time, the student may be doing T'ai Chi Chih one day and suddenly notice that nobody is doing anything, that T'ai Chi Chih is doing T'ai Chi Chih. (This first happened to me in a Japanese garden, and it is a joyous experience.)

Thirdly, after some years of practice one may notice that he or she can do the form mentally. With eyes closed one can visualize the movements and will feel the flow of the Chi, the Vital Force, just as though there were physical movements. So you can be sitting on a plane or attending a boring lecture and, with eyes closed, be enjoying T'ai Chi Chih. This will take considerable time and faithfulness in practice.

To say that practice, preferably daily practice—early in the morning seems the best time, but some people also do it late in the afternoon—is necessary is to point out the obvious. But that practice must be done softly and continuously, preferably at a slow pace. If you rush you will cut the movements short. The "yinning" and "yanging," the bending of the knees and the shift of weight to the bent knee (a slow, steady shift) is all-important, but it must be done softly and evenly.

To sum up: softness at all times, slow and even movements, and no effort; these comprise the "musts" of T'ai Chi Chih movements. Try to observe them at all times.

Forward-Back Foot Positions

When we put a left or right foot forward, the "yinning" and "yanging" (pronounced "yahning") of the feet is shown in the photos. The back heel lifts off the ground as the weight shifts forward, then the front toes rise as the weight shifts to the back leg. These positions apply only to the front-back movements. See "Carry the Ball to the Side" (p. 48) for a description of the sideways "T'ai Chi step" and how it applies to movements having a side-to-side foot position.

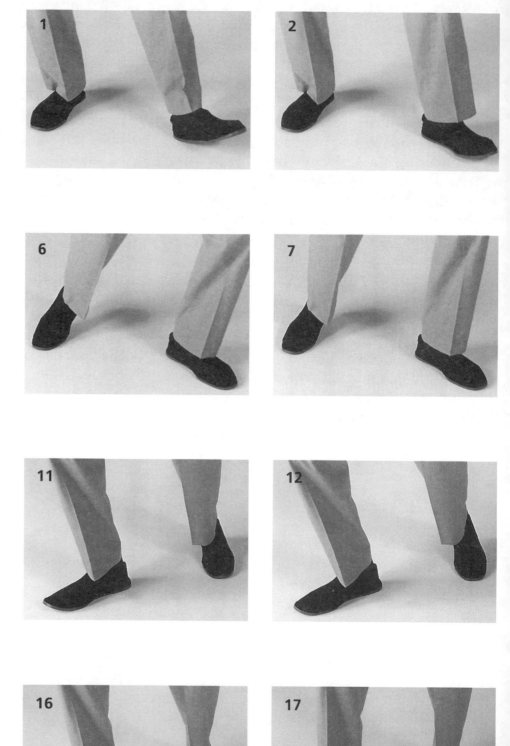

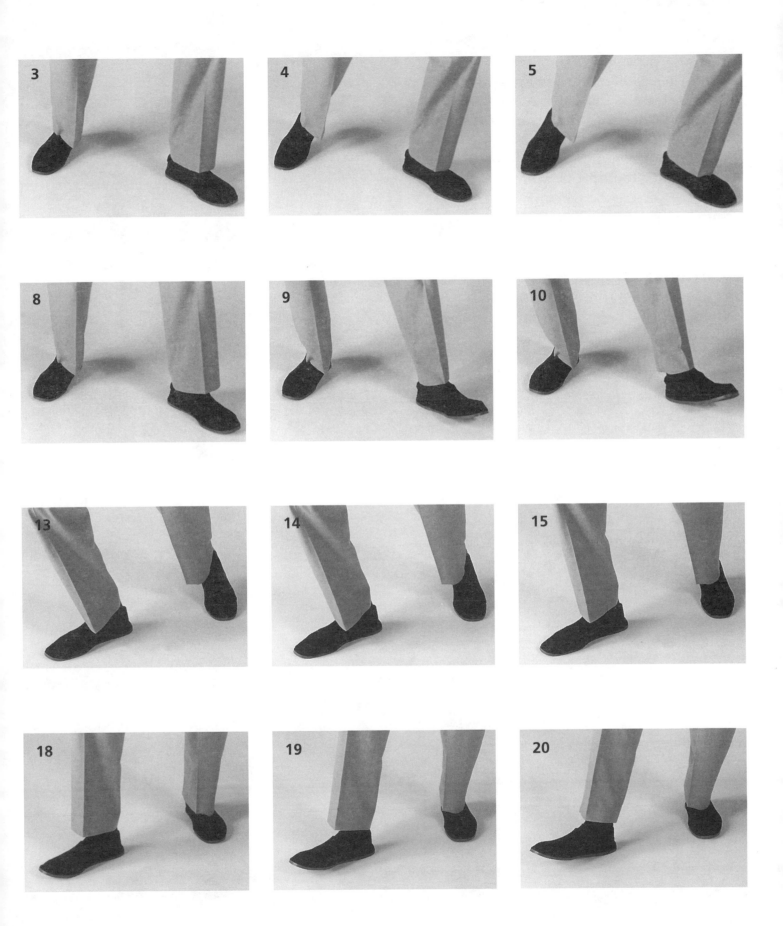

Rocking Motion

As the arms elevate, we rise up on the toes. As the arms descend, we come down flat on the feet, then lift the toes. (Rocking back on the heels can result in losing one's balance.) We usually do this 9 times, 18 times, or 36 times, generally in a multiple of 9.

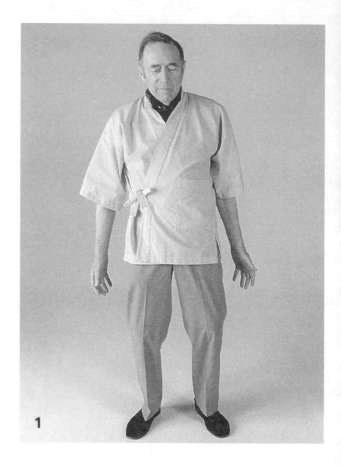

1

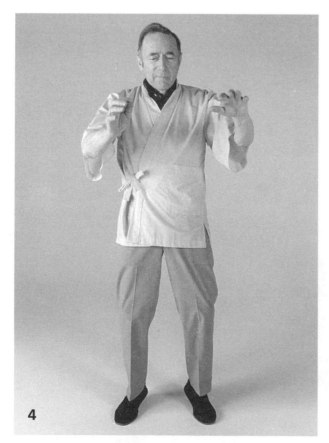

4

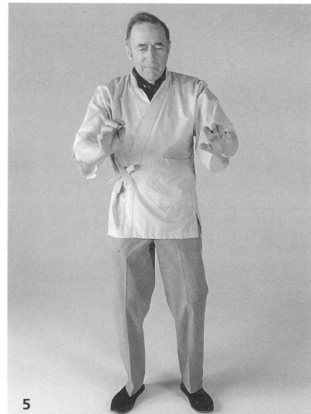

5

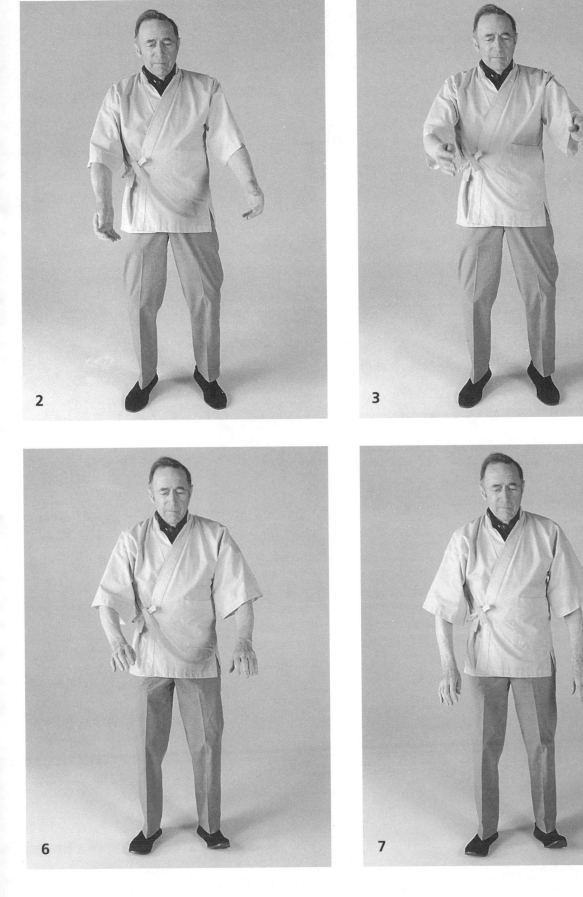

Bird Flaps its Wings

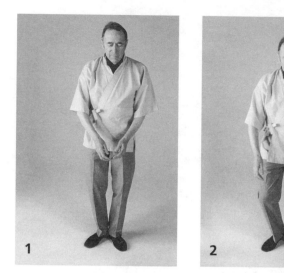

1

2

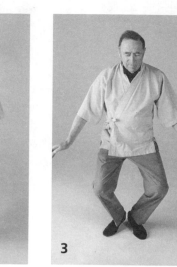

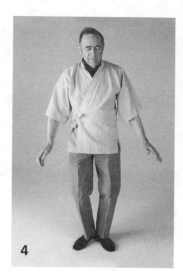

3

4

We do the above sequence twice, heels coming off the ground at Figure 3.

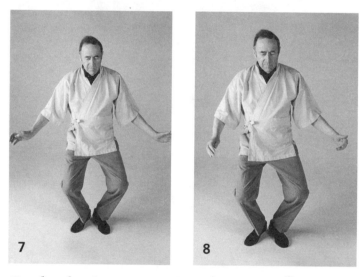

7

8

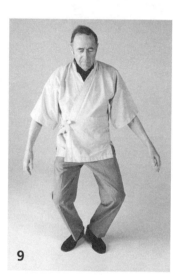

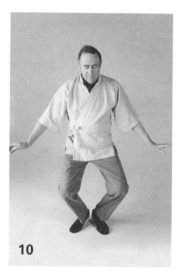

9

10

On the third sequence (Figures 7-12), we do one full circle with the wrists, knees bent. Then from the top of a second circling of the wrists (1½ circles actually), hands slowly come together again, back to the starting position with knees straightened, to repeat the entire set of 3 sequences.

We do these 3 sequences (Figures 1-6 twice, then Figures 7-12) 3 times—or 3 sets of 3.

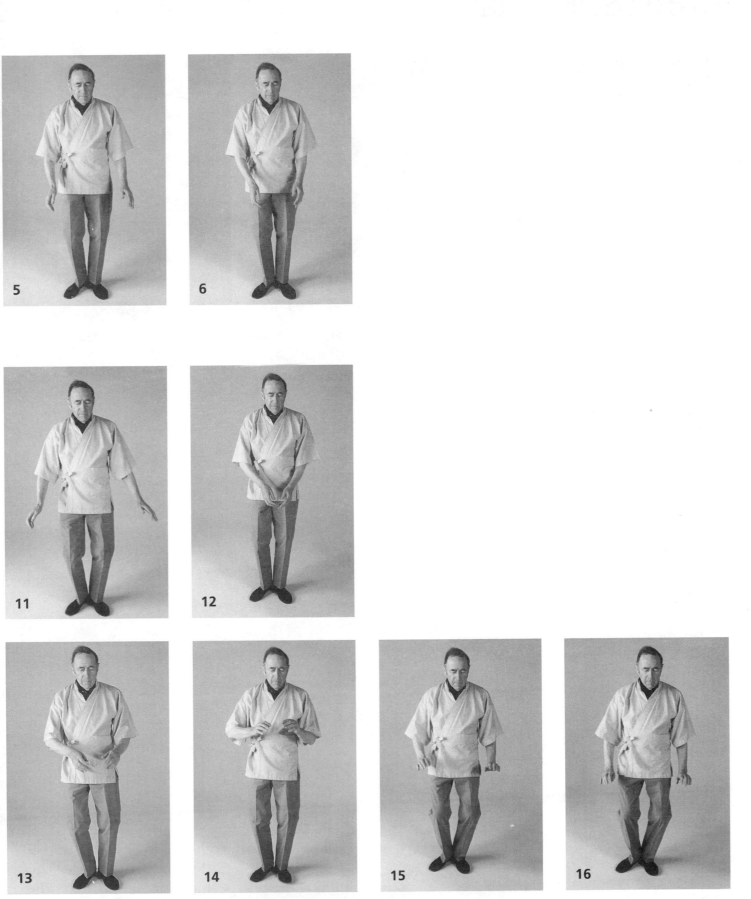

To close, after the hands are together, we raise the arms nearly to the chest, then lower them to the sides, (not to the front), in the graceful finishing pose, knees slightly bent.

Around the Platter (left)

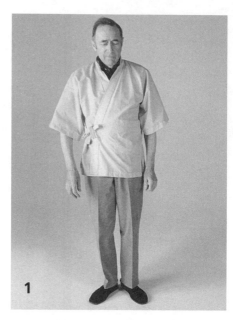

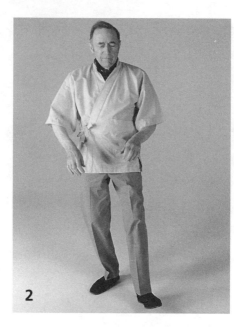

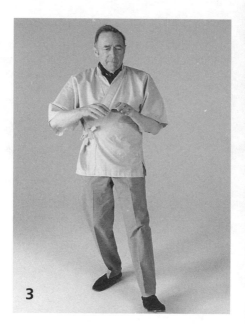

As we lift the arms, we rock back on the right heel and raise the left toes. As we begin to circle the hands (fingers slightly open), we move the weight forward (torso from the waist is held straight up) and gradually shift the weight to the front foot. As we do this very important weight shift entirely to the left foot (yinning and yanging), the right heel gradually raises and the back leg stiffens (straightens). As the hands move past the middle point of the circle, the weight begins to shift back, the rear leg bends and the left toes slowly raise. We do the movement 9 or 18 times.

After we have completed the desired number of circles, we finish as shown in Figures 9 and 10, stepping back, slightly bending the knees and holding the rest position for 15 or 20 seconds to let the yang (positive) and yin (negative) energies (Chi) flow back together. (They separated at the start of the movement.)

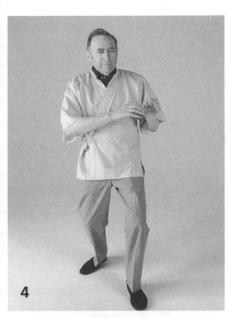

4

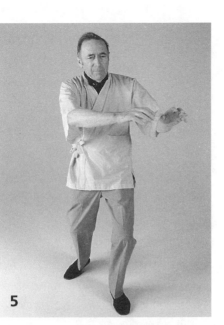

5

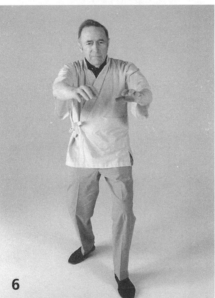

6

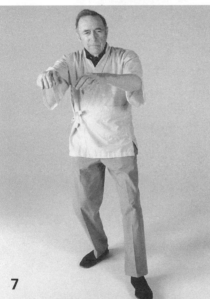

7

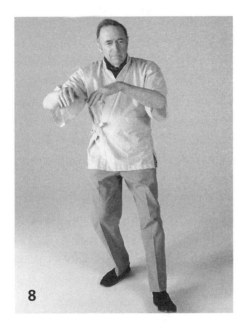

8

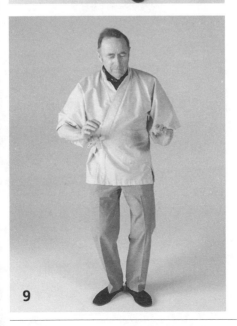

9

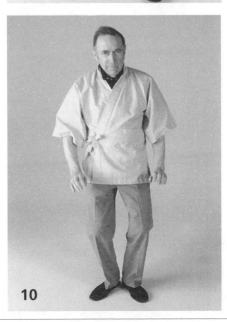

10

Around the Platter (right)

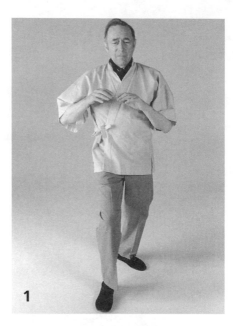

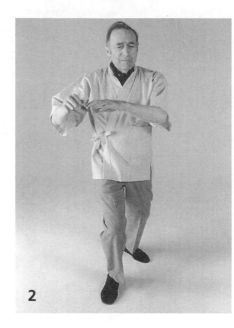

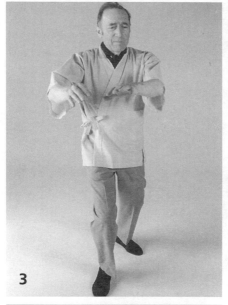

This is the other half of "Around the Platter." From the chest, the arms (hands close together, fingers slightly spread) move to the right and then around in a circle, continuing (without dropping to the side) 9, 18, or any number of times desired. As the weight shifts forward, the back leg stiffens and the back left heel comes off the ground. As the hands return to the chest, we have settled back to where the left leg is bent and the weight rests on it with the right leg straightened and right toes raised (as at the beginning).

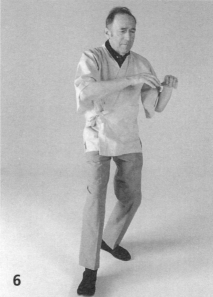

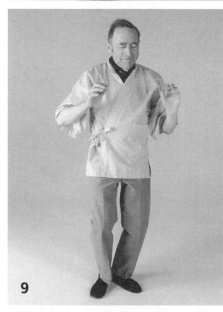

After 9, 18, or 36 circles, we step back so the feet are together. The hands return to the chest, then drop gently down to the closing position, where knees are bent, hand spread with palms down and parallel to the ground (Figures 9-12).

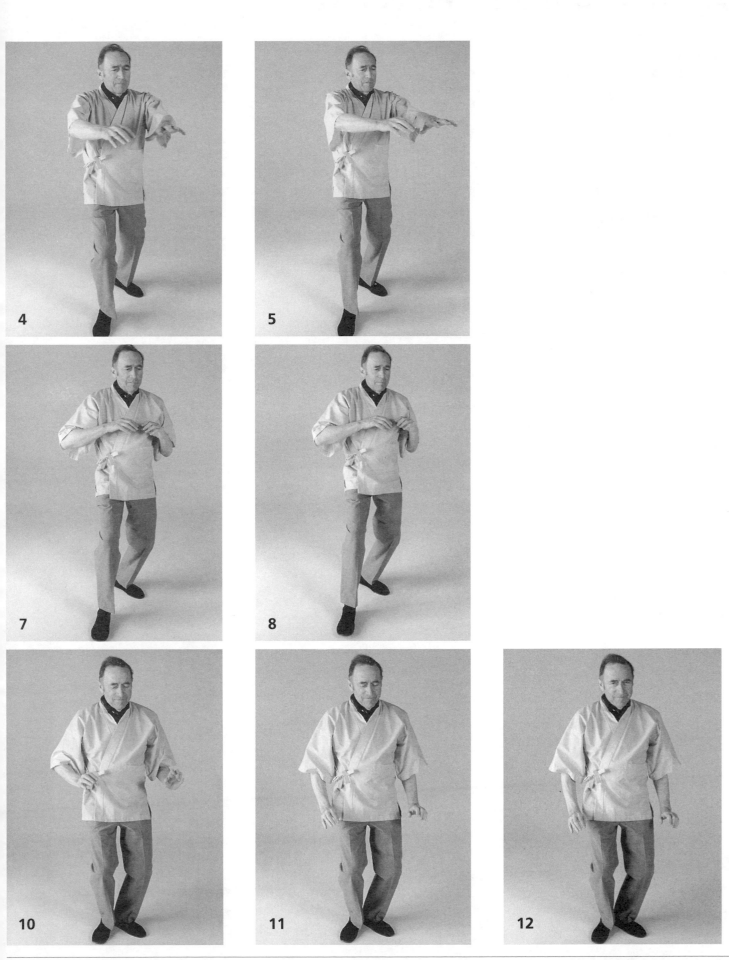

Around the Platter Variation (left)

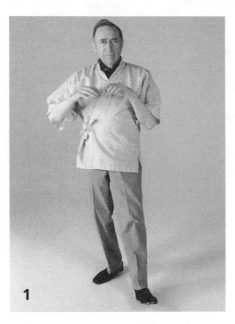

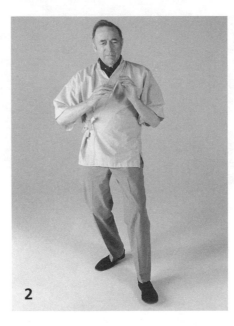

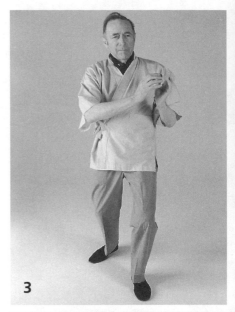

1

2

3

As the hands move left and the weight begins to shift forward, the hands move to cradle a ball (Figure 2) and are held that way until they reach the halfway point in the circle. Then the ball drops and the hands flatten to complete the circle. We must remember to raise the right heel as the weight shifts forward and to raise the left toes as the weight shifts backward.

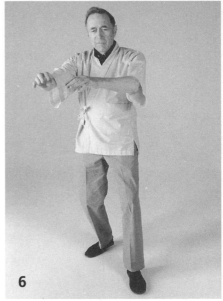

6

After doing 9, 18, or 36 circles (holding the ball till the halfway point), we step back so the feet are together and we lower the hands to a graceful close (Figures 9-11) and relax in this position for 15 to 20 seconds.

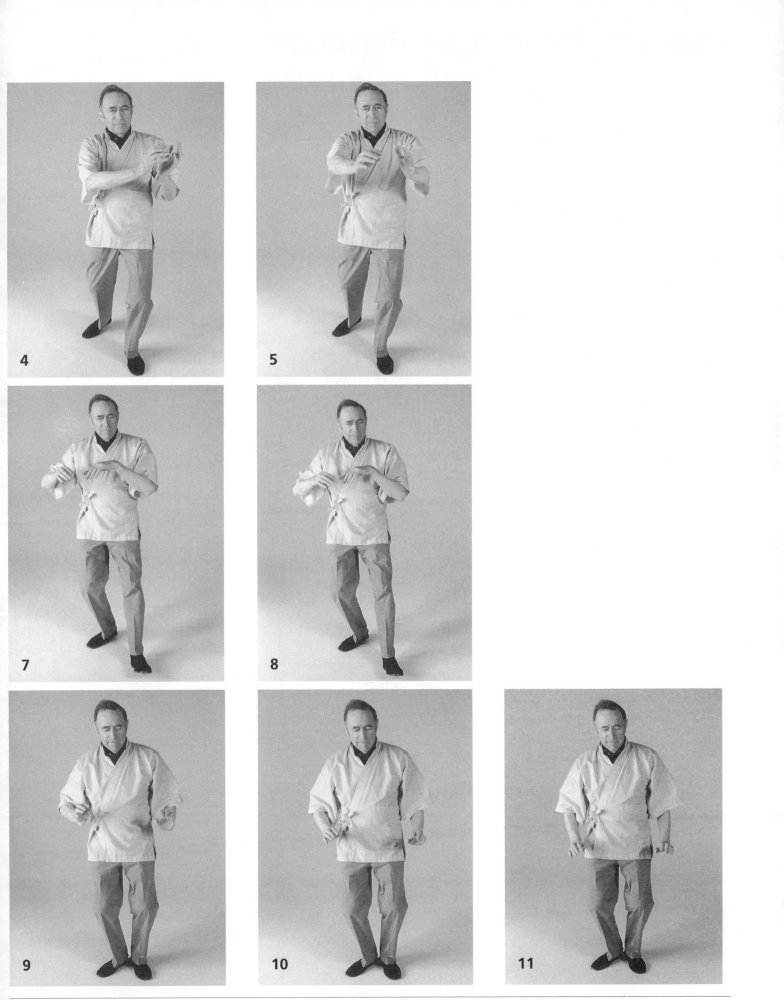

Around the Platter Variation (right)

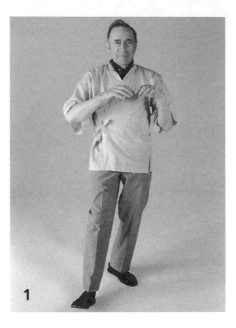

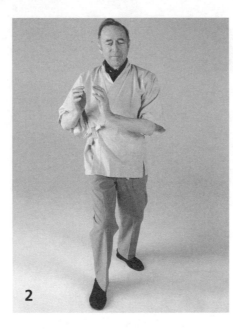

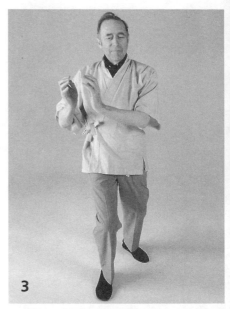

As the hands circle right and begin to cradle a ball, weight shifts forward. At the halfway point, the ball drops and the circle continues back to the starting point at the chest. We do this 9, 18, or 36 times.

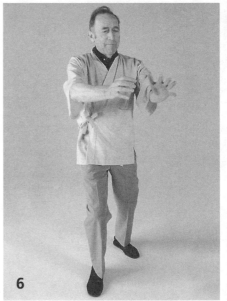

After repeating the movement the desired number of times, from the chest position we gently drop the hands to the sides as we step back, and knees are slightly bent.

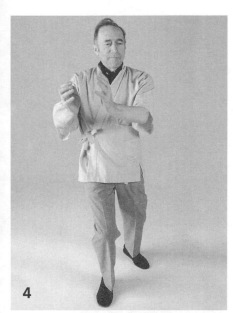

4

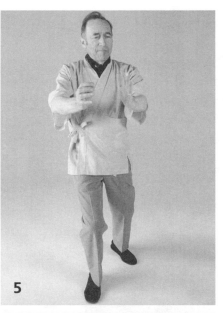

5

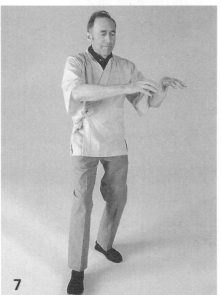

7

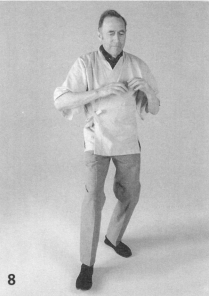

8

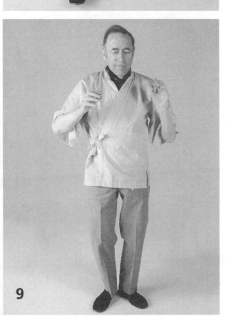

9

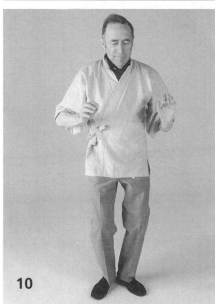

10

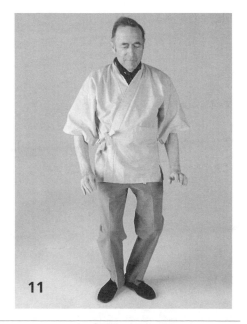

11

Bass Drum (left)

As we begin to rock forward (and heel is raised as weight shifts), we keep the hands, fingers slightly spread, about a foot apart. We imagine we have a bass drum at the chest, and we come down and under it, circling the outside until we are back at the chest position, weight again on the back foot, left toes raised.

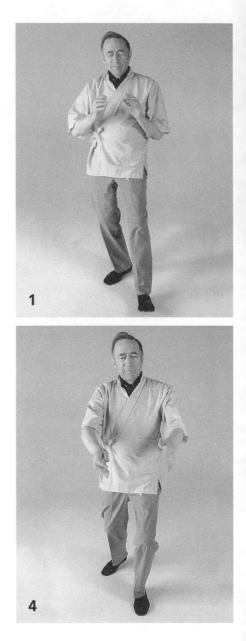

After circling 9 or 18 times, wrists loose and pliable, we step back and drop the hands gently from the chest position and then come to a graceful close with the knees bent.

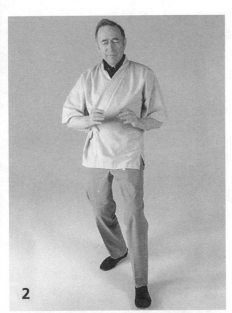

2

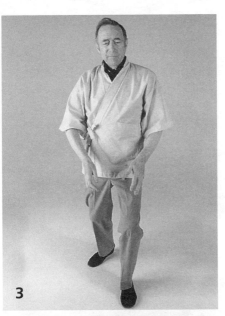

3

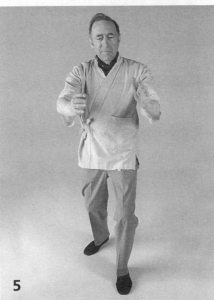

5

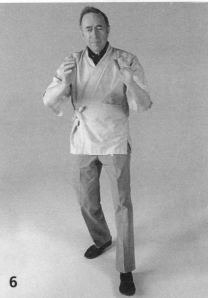

6

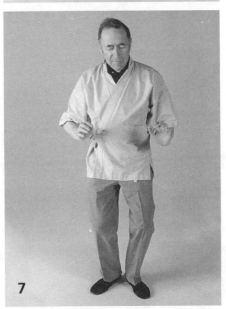

7

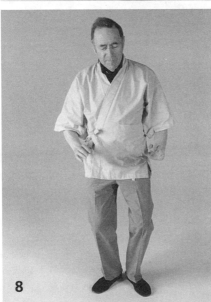

8

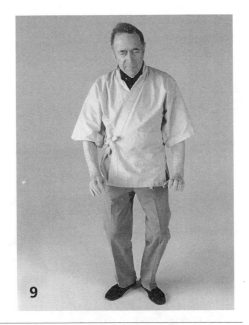

9

Bass Drum (right)

This is the same as "Bass Drum (left)," only the right leg is forward.

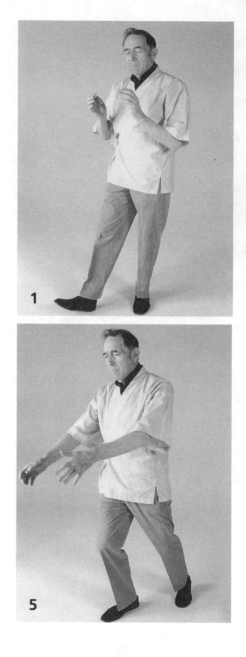

After we do the movement 9 or 18 times, we close as in Figures 8-10. We want to be sure to hold the closing posture (repose) for at least 15 to 20 seconds.

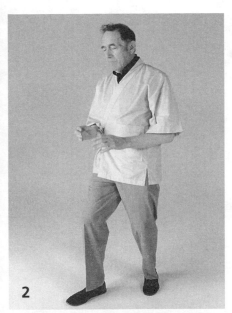

2

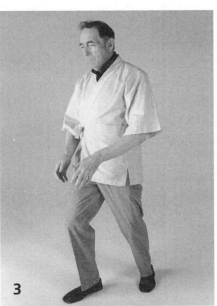

3

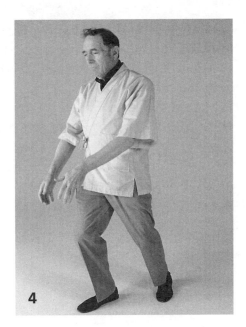

4

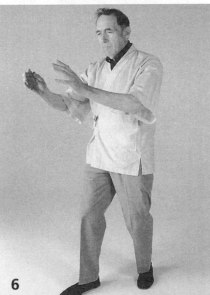

6

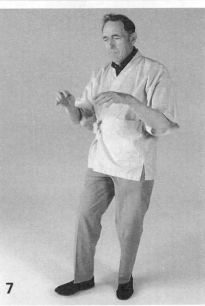

7

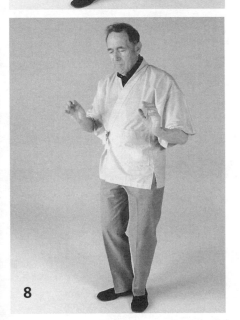

8

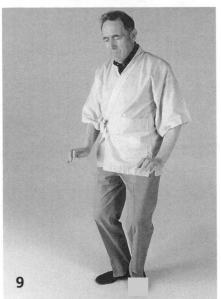

9

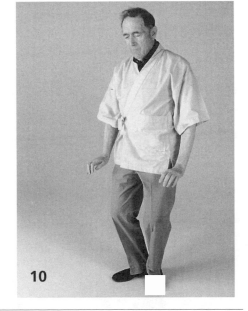

10

Daughter on the Mountaintop (left)

We start low with the hands, as we are going high. As the hands swing wide, toward the top crossing (right hand outside left hand), the weight gradually shifts to the front and the right heel comes off the ground, the right leg stiffening. After the wrists cross (Figure 6), the hands come down and we shift the weight back, but the fingertips remain pointing upward. We do this movement 9, 18, or 36 times.

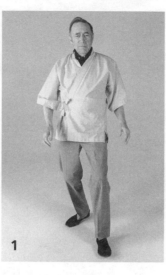

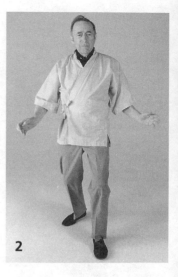

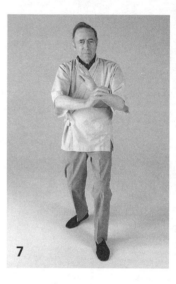

After doing the movement the desired number of times, the hands come up (Figure 12), then down to the sides in the closing posture as we step back so the feet are together.

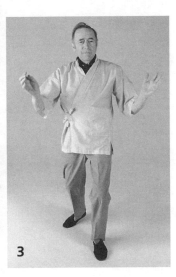

3

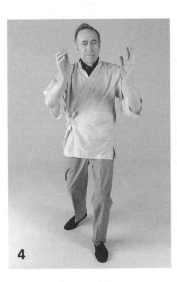

4

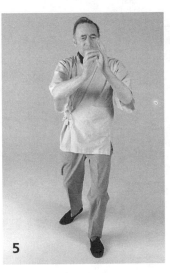

5

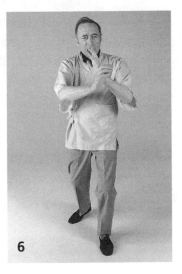

6

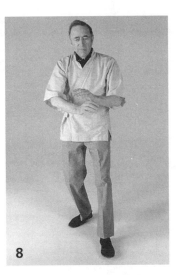

8

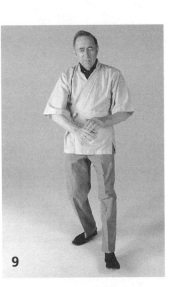

9

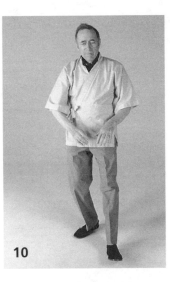

10

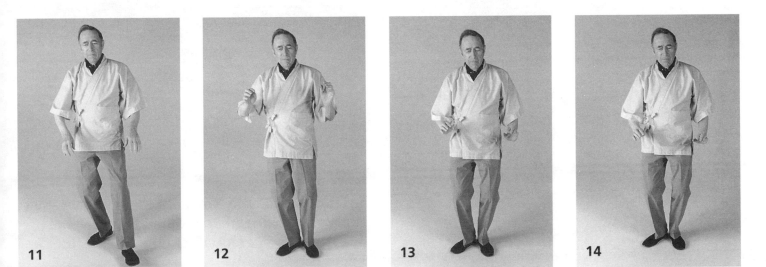

11

12

13

14

Daughter on the Mountaintop (right)

This is the same as "Daughter on the Mountaintop (left)," only the right foot is forward. The right hand *still* passes outside the left hand (no change from the other half of the movement).

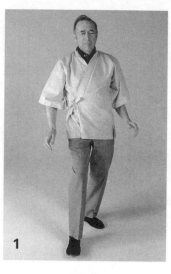

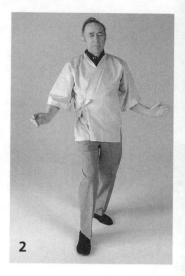

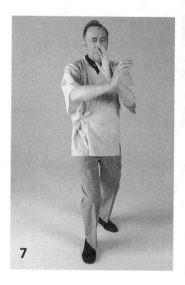

After doing the movement 9, 18, or 36 times, we bring the feet together and hands up (Figure 12), then down gradually to the sides as the knees bend slightly.

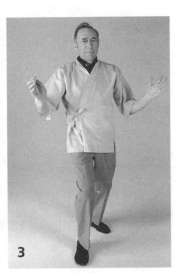

3

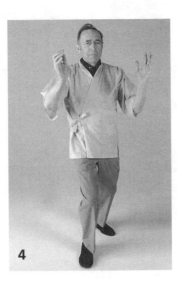

4

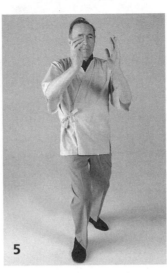

5

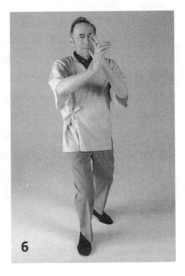

6

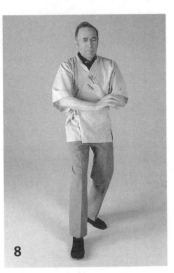

8

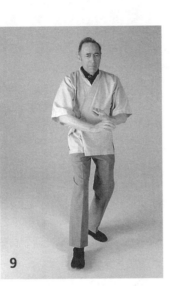

9

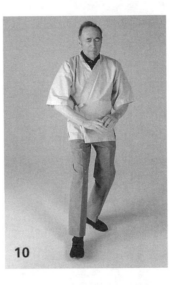

10

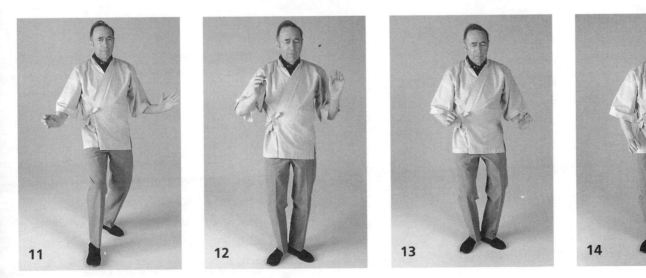

11

12

13

14

Daughter in the Valley (left)

We start high with the hands because we are going low. As the hands come up from the bottom, they are parallel, palms facing each other. The weight keeps moving forward until we reach the top of the arc (Figure 9) and the hands swing wide (Figure 10), before beginning the next downward arc. As in previous movements, we shift the weight forward, then back with the heel rising, then toes rising. The back leg stiffens as the weight moves forward.

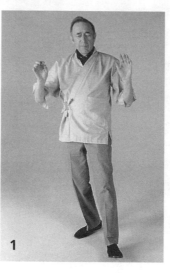

1

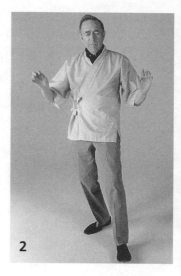

2

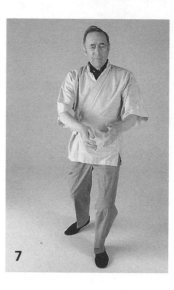

7

After doing the movement the desired number of times, the feet come together and the hands are slightly apart at the shoulder, from which they gradually come down to the rest pose, knees slightly bent.

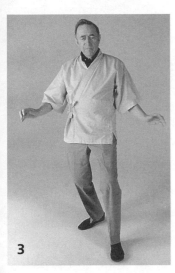

3

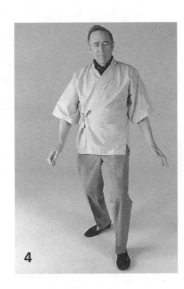

4

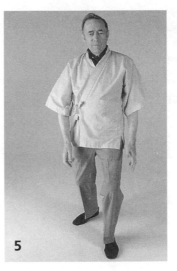

5

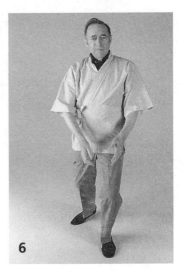

6

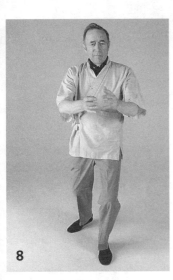

8

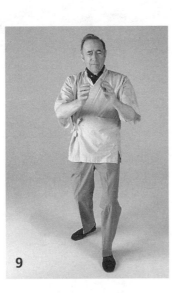

9

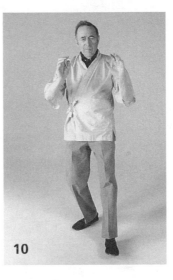

10

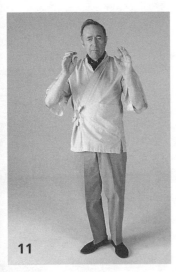

11

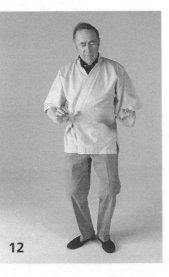

12

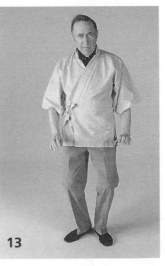

13

Daughter in the Valley (right)

This is the same as "Daughter in the Valley (left)," only the right foot is forward. The weight shift is all-important. Equally important is softness of the hands, with supple wrists, throughout. We do the movement 9, 18, or 36 times.

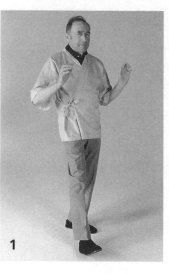 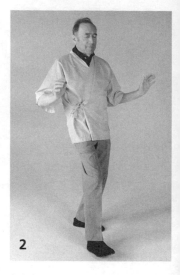

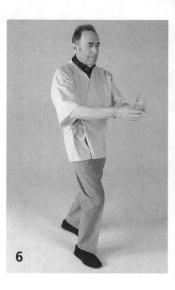

After performing the movement the desired number of times, we bring the feet together and lower both hands to the position of repose, with knees slightly bent.

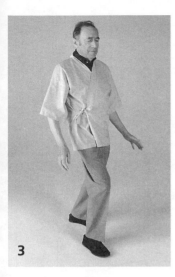

3

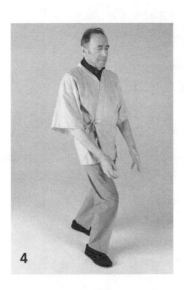

4

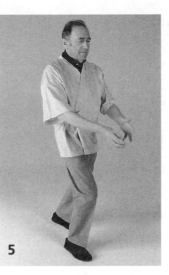

5

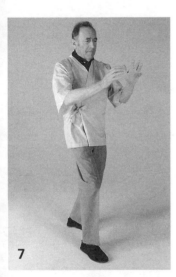

7

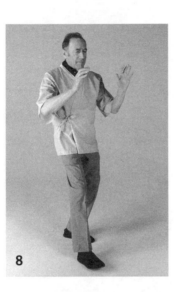

8

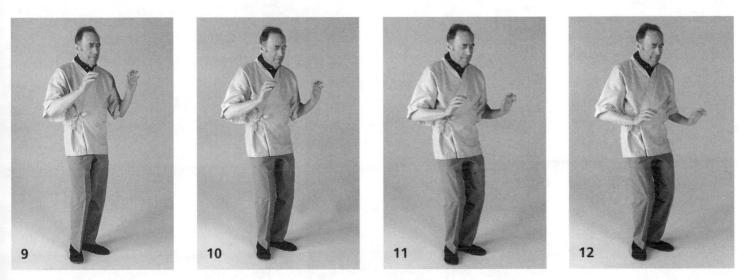

9

10

11

12

Carry the Ball to the Side (left)

Leave plenty of space to the left, as we step to that direction 3 times, moving farther to the left each time.

Here, for the first time, we use the sideways "T'ai Chi step." The left foot lifts slightly off the ground, the knee bends a little, and the foot slithers out slightly, landing on the heel and quickly flattening.

As the weight shifts to the left (not too markedly), the hands carry the ball, circling past the general area of the waist and continue in a circle. (One circle is pictured in Figures 2-10.) The hands make 3 circles in all, with the weight shifting back and forth until finally, the right leg moves over to the left leg (Figure 11) and the hands come down to the position of rest (Figure 12).

We rest (a few seconds) and then step to the left from our new position and do 3 more circles before coming to rest (Figures 1-12).

A third time, we step to the left, meaning we have moved 3 times in that direction, do 3 circles with the hands, and come to a position of rest. Thus, we have a movement of 3 times 3.

From here we will move back to the right (see pp. 50-51).

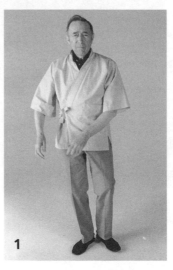

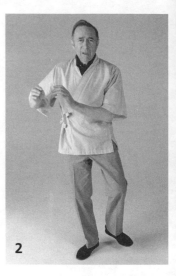

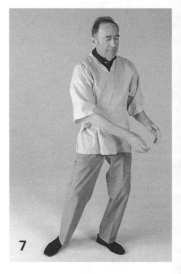

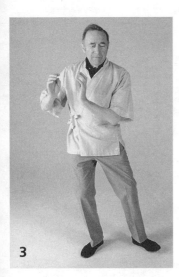

3

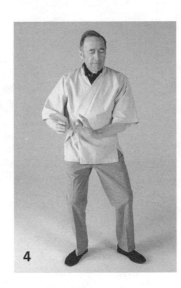

4

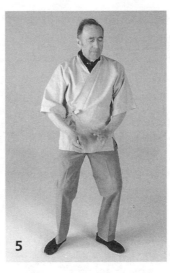

5

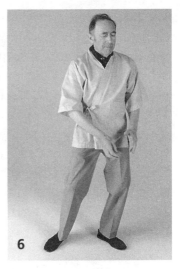

6

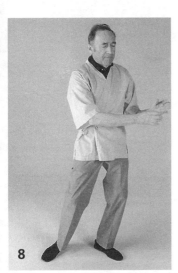

8

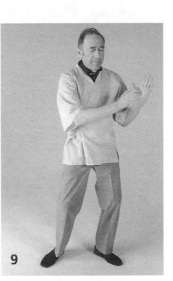

9

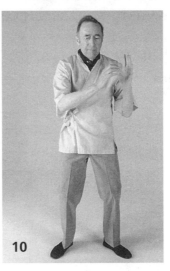

10

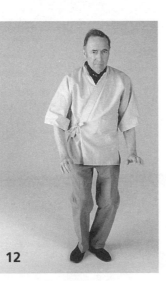

11

12

Carry the Ball to the Side (right)

We now move to the right, reversing what we did in "Carry the Ball to the Side (left)" so that we finish the entire sequence in the same spot where we began. After making 3 circles and shifting the weight back and forth (Figures 1-11), we take the rest position (Figures 12-13). Then we begin again, taking a step to the right, doing 3 circles to the right, bringing the feet together, and taking the position of repose. One more time we step to the right (T'ai Chi step) and circle 3 times with the hands, to take the final position of rest where we started.

As we step to the right, we emphasize the left hand slightly. When we originally stepped to the left, we emphasized the right hand slightly. The bent leg (with weight on it) is yang, so we emphasize the opposing hand to balance, as the stronger hand is also yang. We do not need to be too concerned about this emphasis.

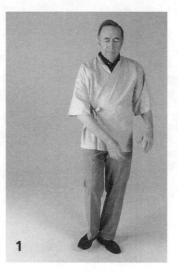

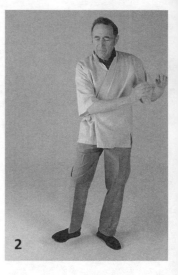

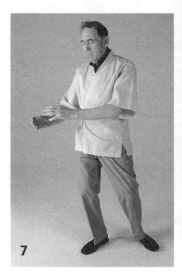

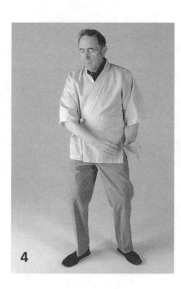

3

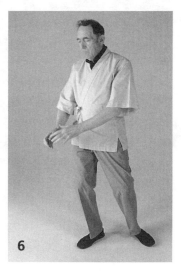

4

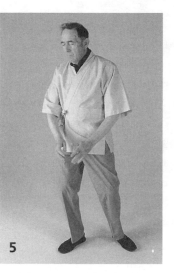

5

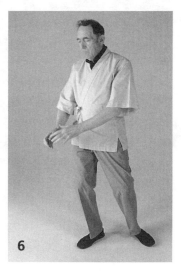

6

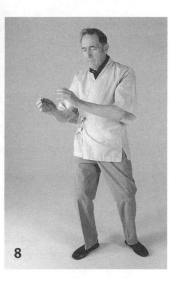

8

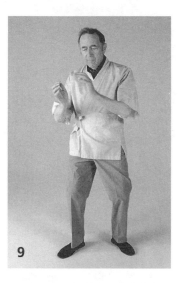

9

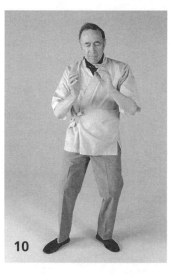

10

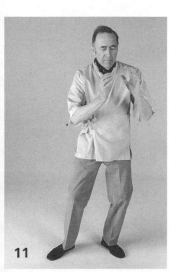

11

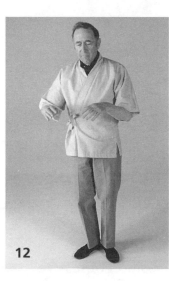

12

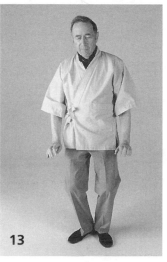

13

Push Pull (left)

As the weight shifts to the front foot (back heel coming off the ground), we slightly emphasize the right hand to balance the positive left foot. It is important to note that the hands do not push directly forward but dip slightly ⌣ . Then we turn the palms up as we begin to pull back, up and over ⌢. We emphasize the right hand as we move forward; when moving back, there is no emphasis. We do this movement 9, 18, or 36 times.

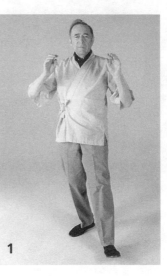

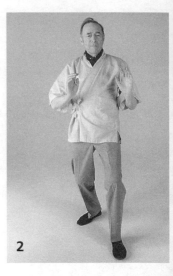

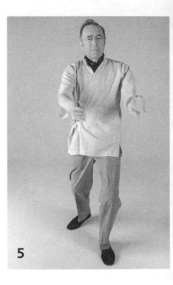

After the desired number of repetitions, the feet come together and we begin to lower the hands (and slightly bend the knees) in the position of rest.

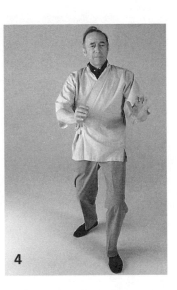

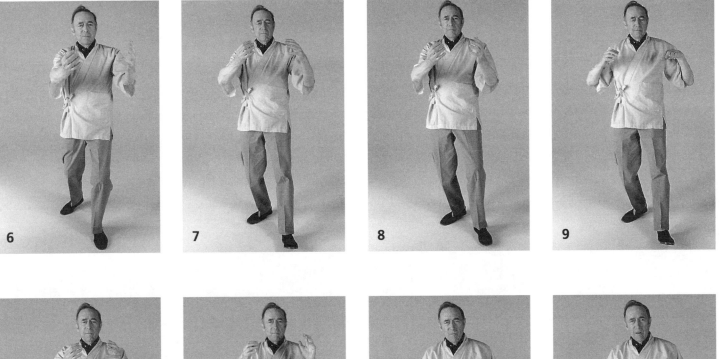

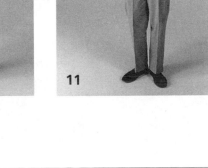

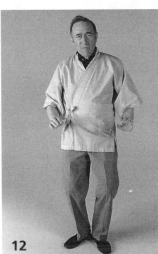

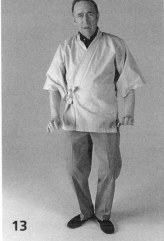

Push Pull (right)

We note how pushing the hands makes a slight dip going forward and a slight rise coming back, forming an elongated circle ⬭. Circularity is all-important in T'ai Chi Chih.

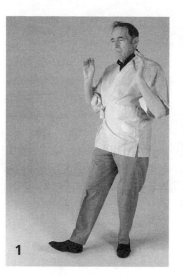 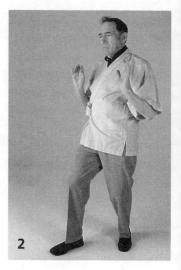

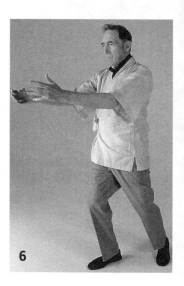

After the desired number of repetitions, the feet come together and we make the gradual hand descent to the position of rest, knees slightly bent.

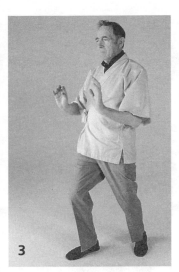

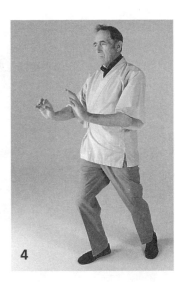

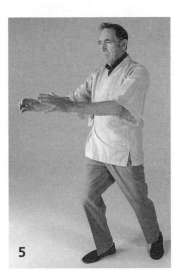

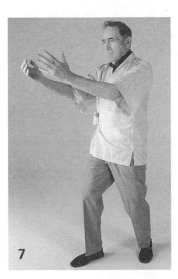

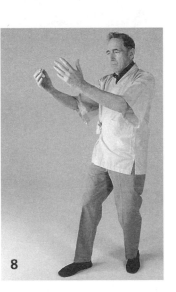

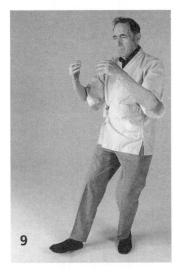

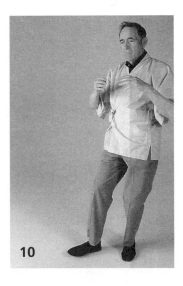

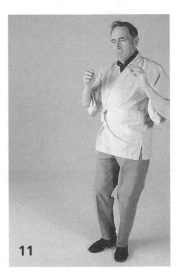

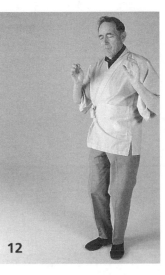

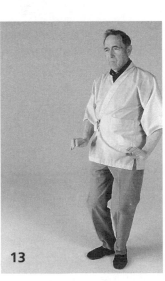

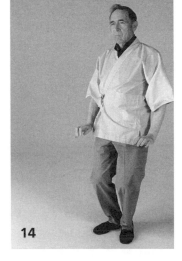

Pulling in the Energy (left)

"Pulling in the Energy" is like "Around the Platter," only the *palms are turned upward*. As we circle the hands from left to right, we visualize the energy from the most distant star coming in through the fingertips. This *visualization* is important.

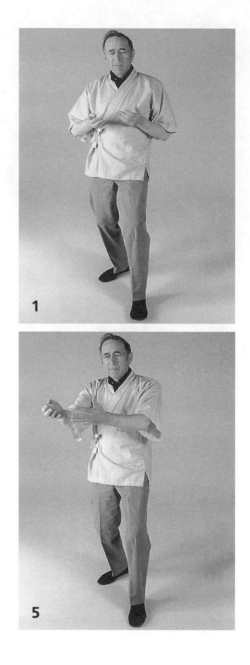

After the desired number of repetitions, we bring the feet together and come down to the position of rest. We must do all movements slowly and evenly, with no tension at all.

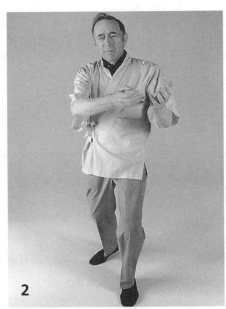

2

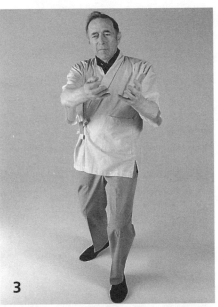

3

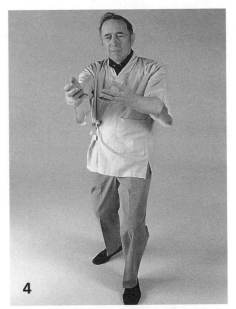

4

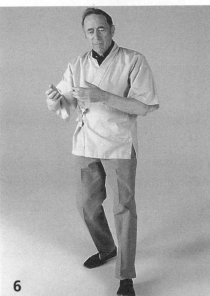

6

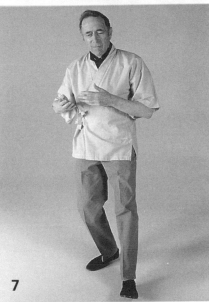

7

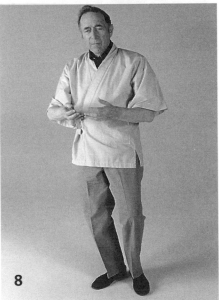

8

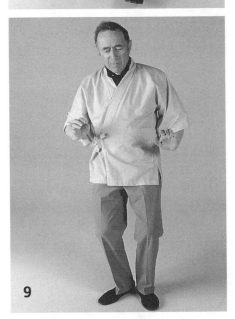

9

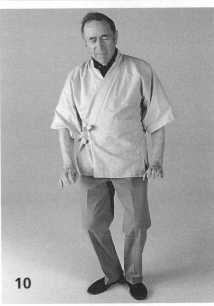

10

Pulling in the Energy (right)

Now we circle to the right, right leg forward. Don't forget the visualization.

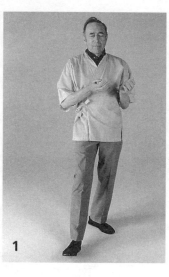
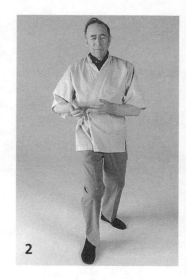

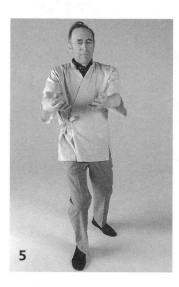

After finishing the desired number of repetitions, we bring the feet together and let the hands descend to the position of repose. We always remember to "swim through the very heavy air, slowly, with no effort."

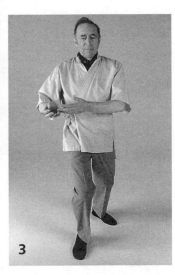

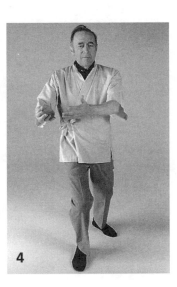

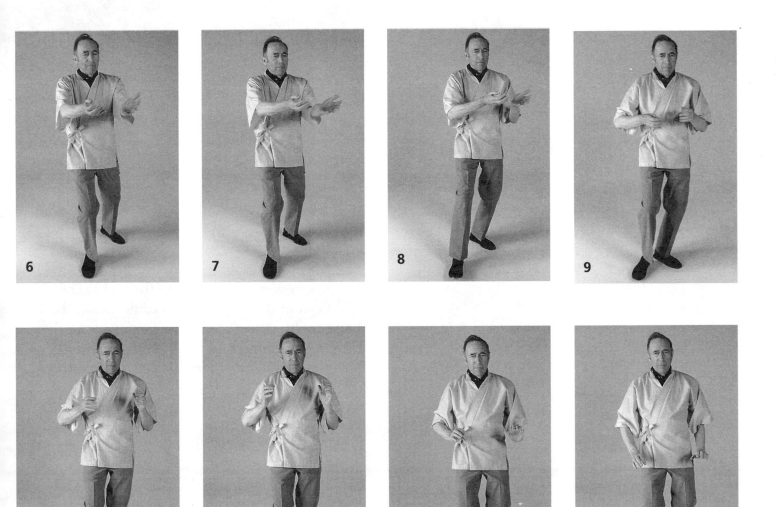

Pulling Taffy (left and right)

As we take the "T'ai Chi step" to the left and gradually shift the weight to that leg, we pull the left hand (palm up) past the right hand, which is on top with the palm facing down. The right hand finishes palm down close to the right leg (Figure 7), which carries no weight, and the left hand (which pulled the "taffy") is facing up to the sun (Figure 7). We come to a position of rest by bringing the insubstantial right leg to join the left.

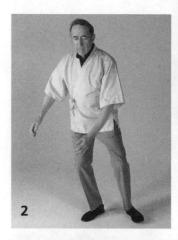

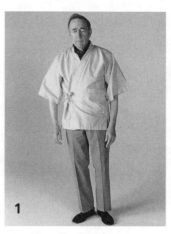

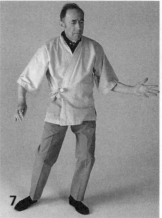

We now reverse the move to the right. The right hand (palm up) pulls across underneath the left hand (palm down) as the weight shifts to the right leg. We finish in the position of repose by bringing the insubstantial left leg to join the right.

We can do the whole routine, left and right, continuously 3, 6, or 9 times. We do not stand with the legs straight at any time in "Pulling Taffy." The legs should be slightly bent and the body slightly lower than normal at all times.

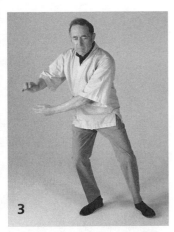

3

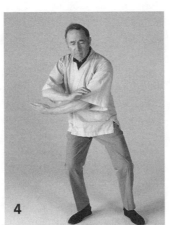

4

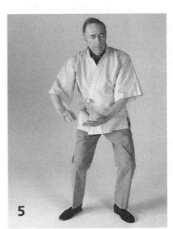

5

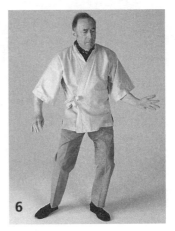

6

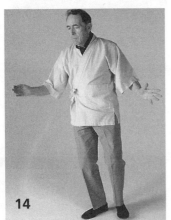

8

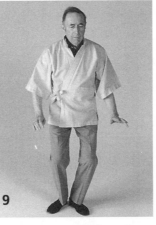

9

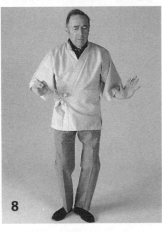

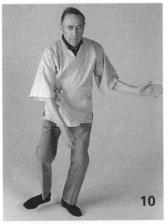

10

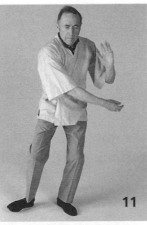

11

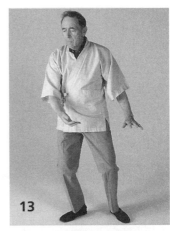

12

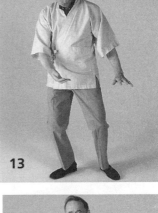

13

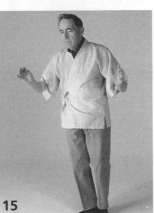

14

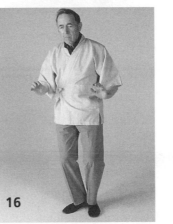

15

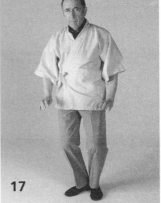

16

17

Pulling Taffy–1st Variation–Anchor (left)

Keeping the back foot anchored (stationary), we turn the body to the right and begin to do "Pulling Taffy" to the front, left leg advanced. After the left hand (palm up) has crossed under the right hand (palm down), we step back as the left hand continues circling, coming to a rest position. Figure 8 shows how the feet come together, a step back with the left foot.

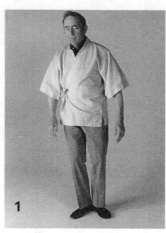

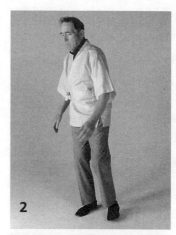

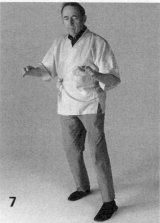

We now do the basic "Pulling Taffy" to the left, coming to a graceful conclusion.

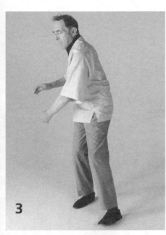

3

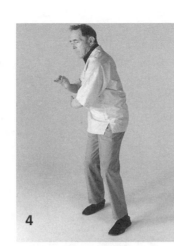

4

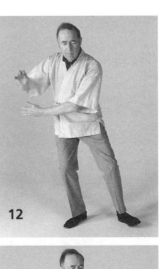

5

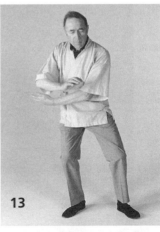

6

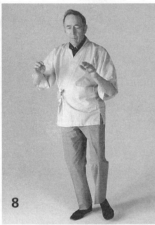

8

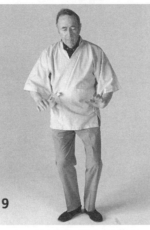

9

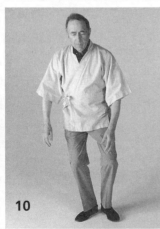

10

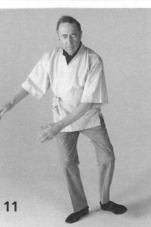

11

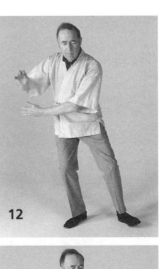

12

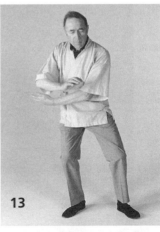

13

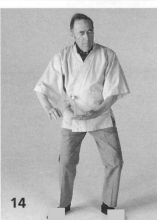

14

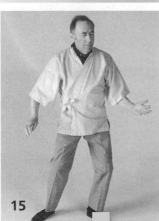

15

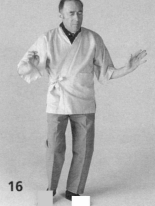

16

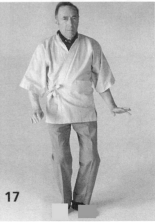

17

Pulling Taffy–1st Variation–Anchor (right)

This time we put the right foot forward, while the left foot remains anchored (we become pigeon-toed). We do "Pulling Taffy" going forward, then pull back to the rest position.

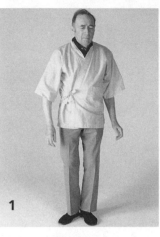

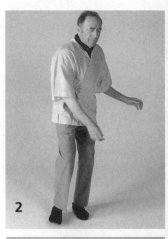

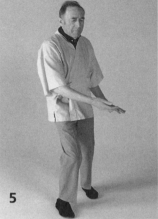

Now we do the basic "Pulling Taffy" to the right. The entire sequence (Figures 1-7 and Figures 8-15) is continuous.

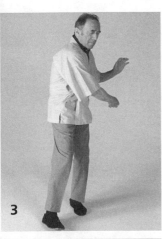

3

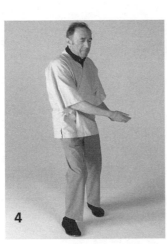

4

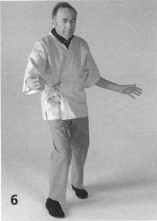

6

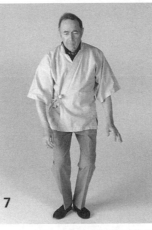

7

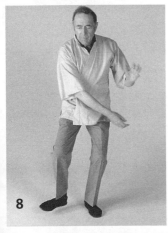

8

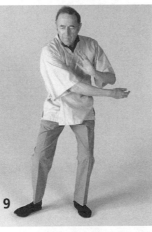

9

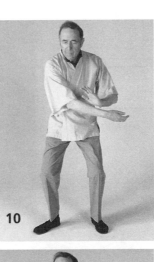

10

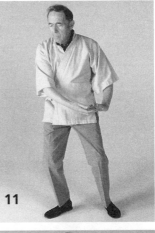

11

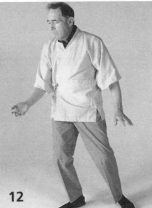

12

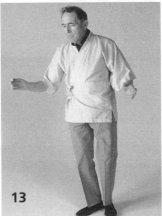

13

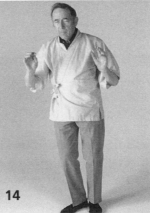

14

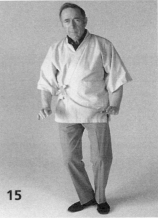

15

Pulling Taffy–2nd Variation–Wrist Circles (left)

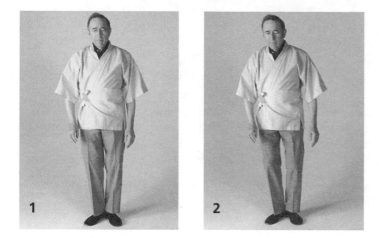

1 **2** **3** **4**

We rise on the toes (heels together), spread the arms, and circle with the wrists 3 times. The heels leave the ground 2 times, and remain flat on the third circling of the wrists.

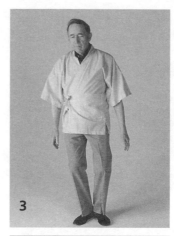

6

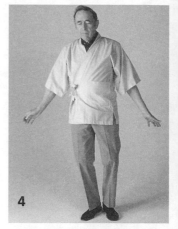

7

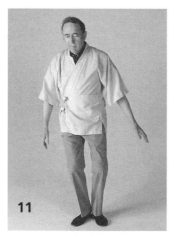

11

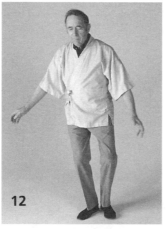

12

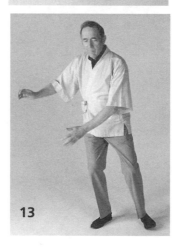

13

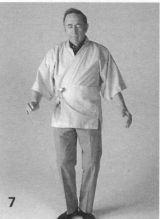

14

We now do the basic "Pulling Taffy" to the left (the entire sequence is continuous), coming to rest in the repose position.

Notice where feet pull together, right foot moving over to the left (Figure 19).

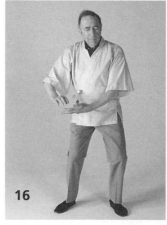

16

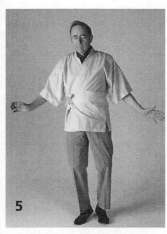

5

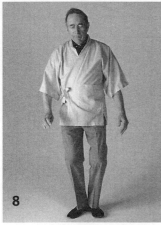

8

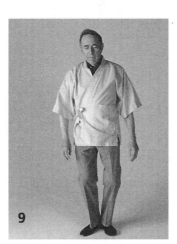

9

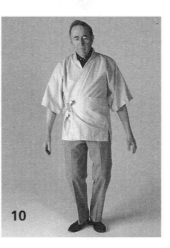

10

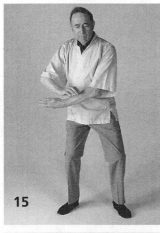

15

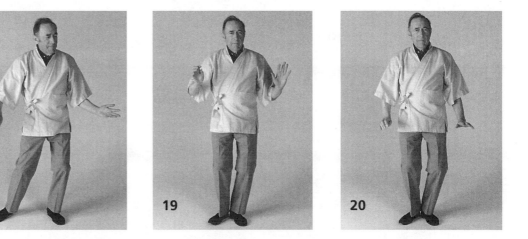

17

18

19

20

Pulling Taffy–2nd Variation–Wrist Circles (right)

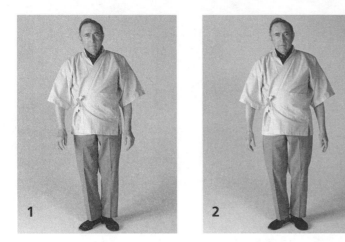

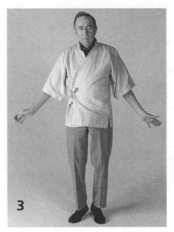

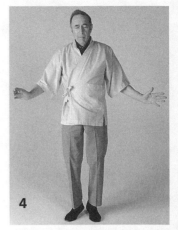

We rise on the toes, move the arms to the sides (simultaneously), and circle the wrists 3 times.

We do not stay on the toes. We come down flat on the feet after each of the first and second wrist circles, then *stay flat* as we begin the third circle.

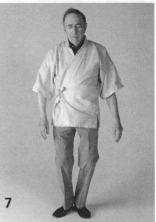

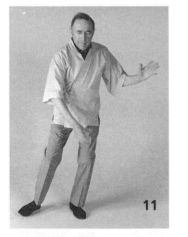

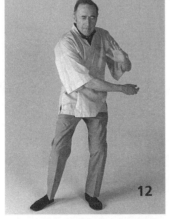

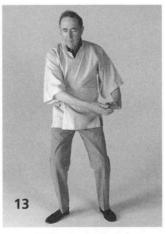

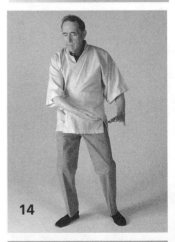

From the *top* of the third circle (Figure 11), we begin the basic "Pulling Taffy" to the right. On the third circle the heels are kept flat on the ground.

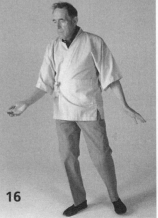

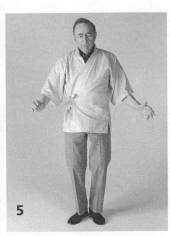

5

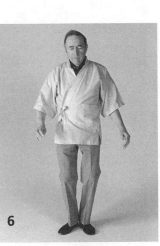

6

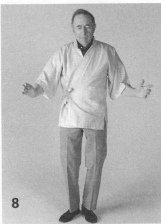

8

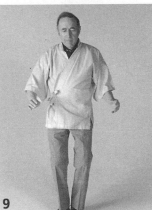

9

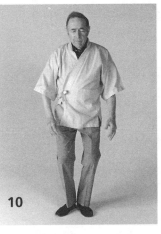

10

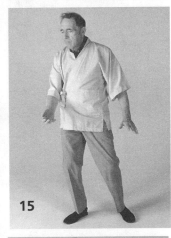

15

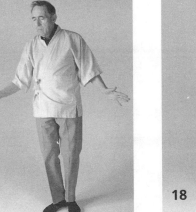

17

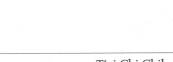

18

Pulling Taffy–3rd Variation–Perpetual Motion

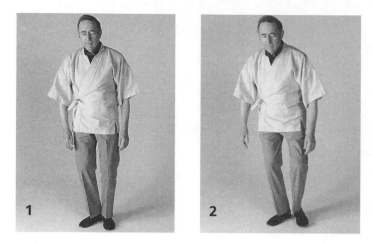

1   2   3   4

We do the basic "Pulling Taffy" to the left, then pull the right hand across (Figure 11) into position to do "Pulling Taffy" to the right (without pause). Figure 19 shows how we get into position to do the second pull to the left. We might do this movement 9 times (continuously), alternating left and right. There is no pause.

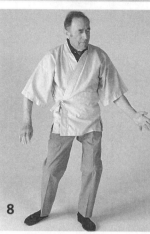

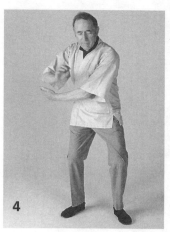

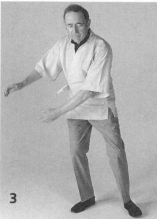

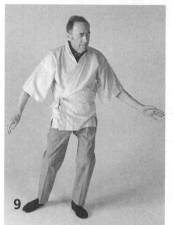

8   9

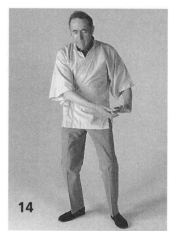

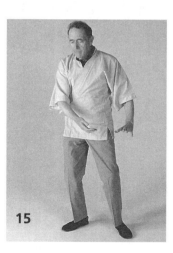

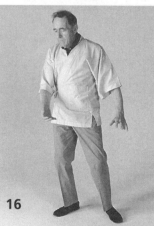

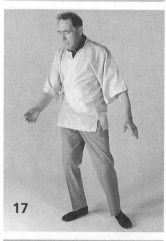

14   15   16   17

Figures 22-26 show how we close to the right, bringing the feet together and coming to the rest position.

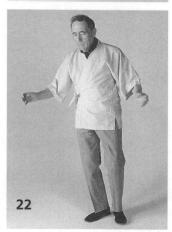

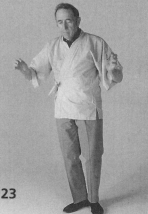

22   23

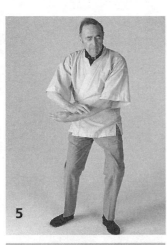 5

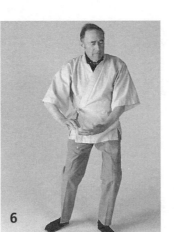 6

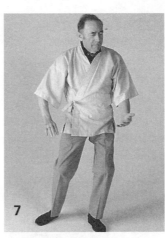 7

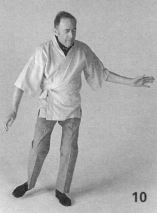 10

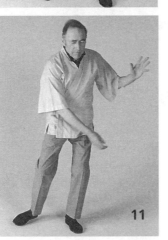 11

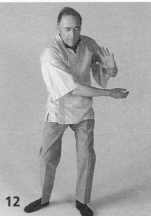 12

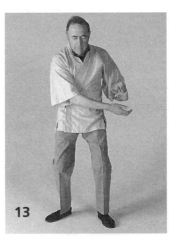 13

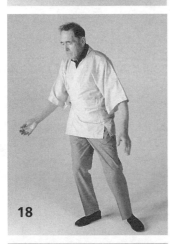 18

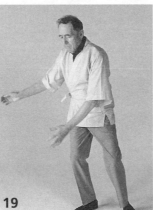 19

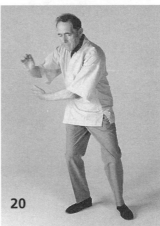 20

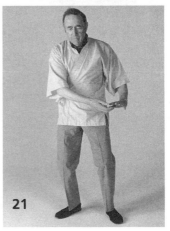 21

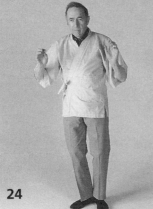 24

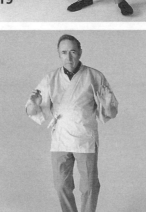 25

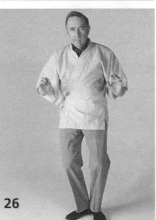 26

Working the Pulley (left)

With the left leg forward, we push out with the left hand, as the right hand comes down slightly below the waist and pulls back, palm up, behind the body. The right hand comes up and over the shoulder (swimming motion) and the left hand pulls back, palm up, about waist level. As the left hand goes behind the body, the right hand is pushed forward and the body *(from the waist only)* is turned to face left (see Figures 8-10). Then the left hand comes up and over and the right hand pulls back. Nine or 18 repetitions are enough.

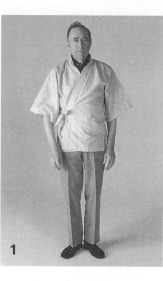

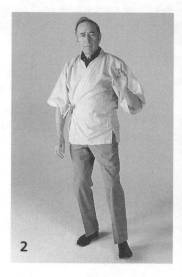

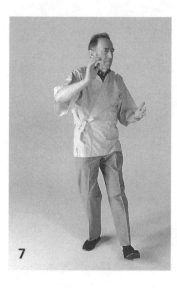

We conclude with the right hand coming up and over the shoulder. That hand pushes forward, the left hand does a modest circle (not up and over the shoulder), and, the feet now together, the two hands come parallel and go down slowly to the rest position, knees slightly bent.

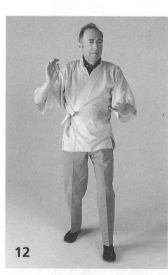

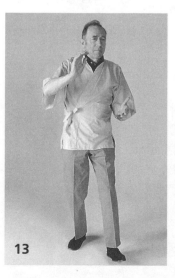

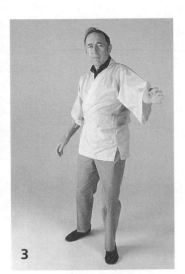

3

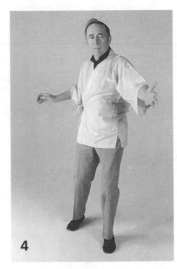

4

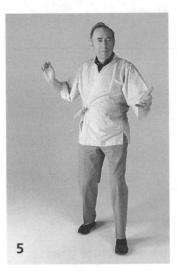

5

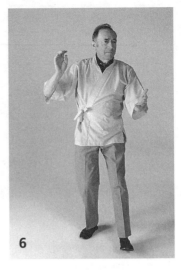

6

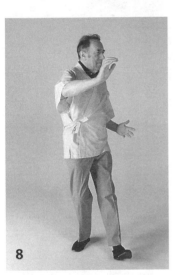

8

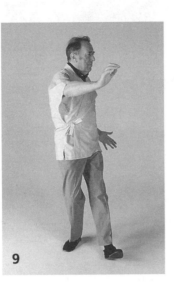

9

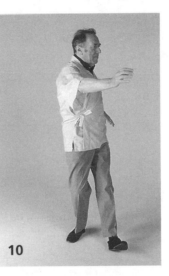

10

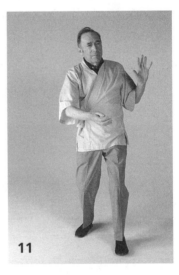

11

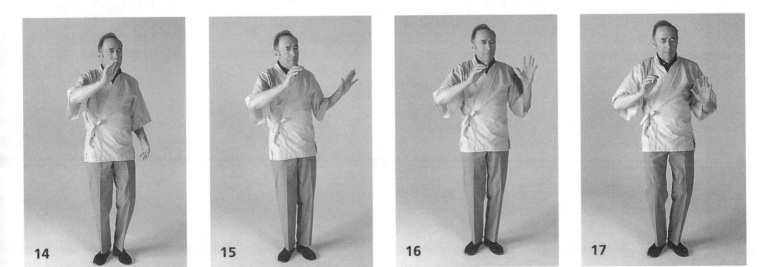

14

15

16

17

Working the Pulley (right)

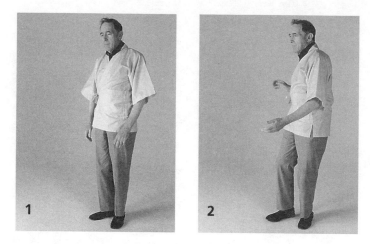

1

2

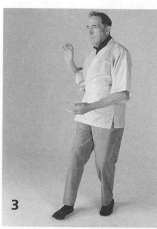

3

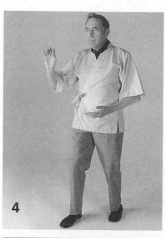

4

We step forward with the right foot as the right hand moves forward from the shoulder. Simultaneously, the left hand pulls back, palm up, then up and over the shoulder as the body *above the waist* turns sharply to the right. Then the left hand, which has pushed out, comes back and the right hand goes up and over the shoulder. We do this movement 9 or 18 times.

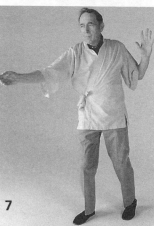

7

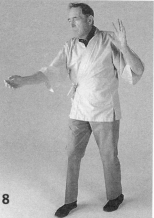

8

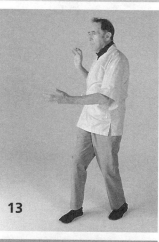

13

After the desired number of repetitions, we finish as pictured in Figures 17-20. It is important to note that the feet come together as the right hand makes a small vertical circle and the two hands come together and proceed to the rest position.

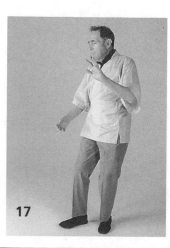

17

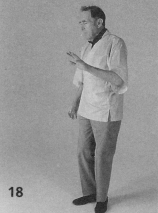

18

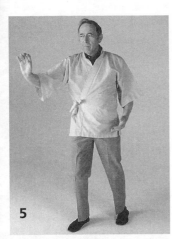

5

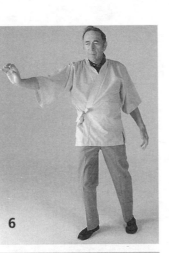

6

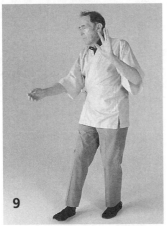

9

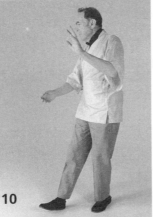

10

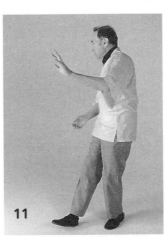

11

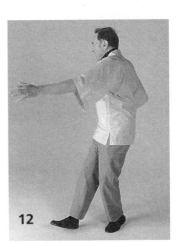

12

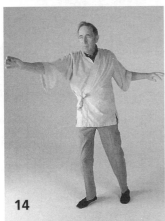

14

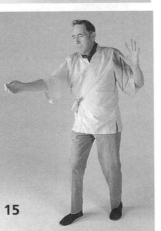

15

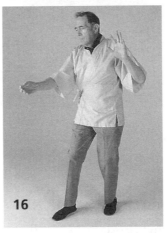

16

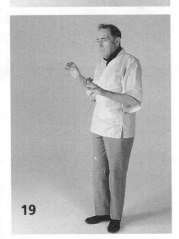

19

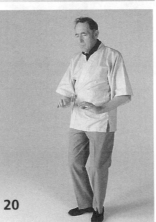

20

Light at the Top of the Head / Light at the

The hands are softly raised to the top of the head, then the wrists flare out as we rise onto the toes. The hands come back to the original position above the head (Figure 6) as we come back flat on the feet. We do this sequence 3 times, followed by a pause of a few seconds as the hands are still (positioned as in Figure 6). They now circle forward slowly for a few seconds, facing each other (forward circles not shown in photos). There is a pause. Then the wrists flare out again 3 times and come down as in Figures 7-11.

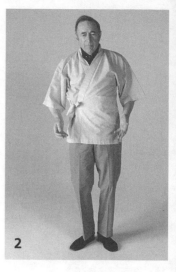

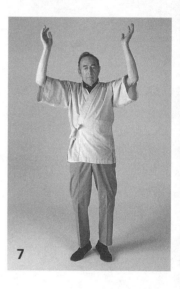

The hands pass at the center (Figure 12), right hand under left, proceed palms up to chest level (Figure 13), turn downward and come down to the position of rest.

"Light at the Temple" can be done the same way as "Light at the Top of the Head," except that the hands are raised to face the temples and flare out from there.

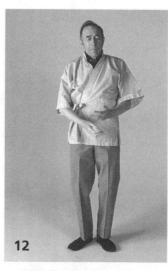

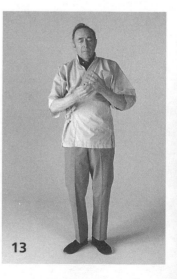

Temple

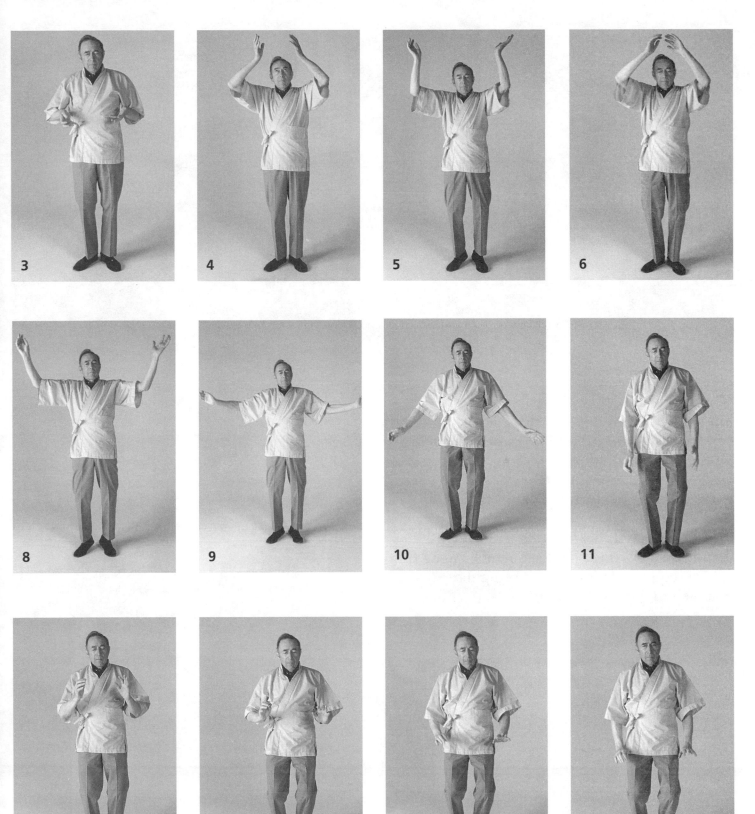

Joyous Breath

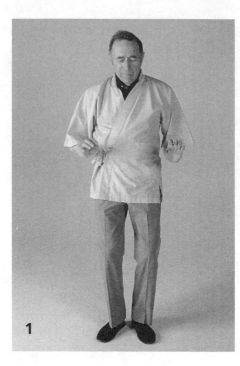

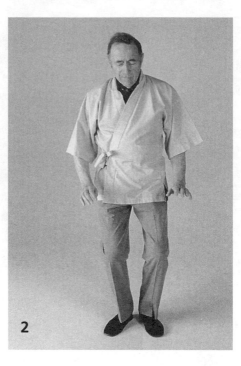

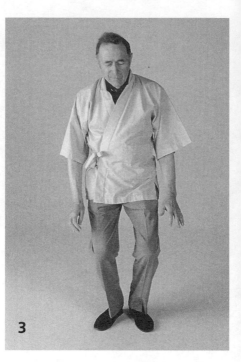

1

2

3

This is the only movement that uses force. Breathing out through the nostrils, we push the air down into the ground, then turn the palms up and breathe in deeply through the nostrils as we pull the arms up to the chest, rising on our toes. We now turn the hands over and push them down toward the ground as our breath flows out in 4 sections, guided by the hands pushing down in 4 segments. We do this entire sequence 3 times, then bring the hands into the rest position.

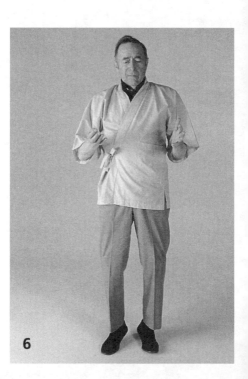

6

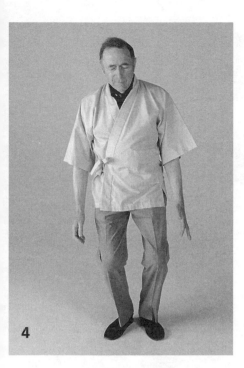

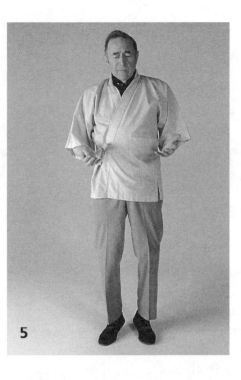

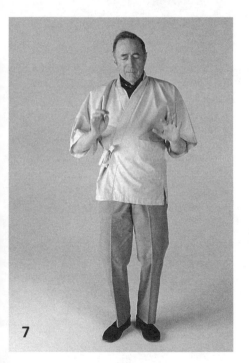

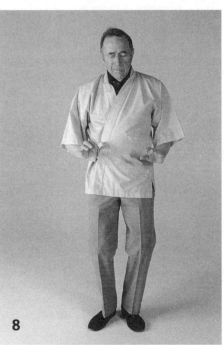

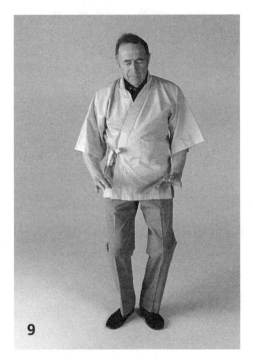

Passing Clouds

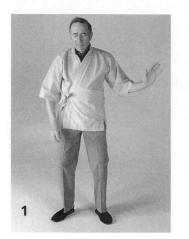 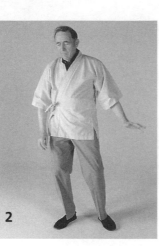 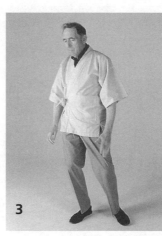 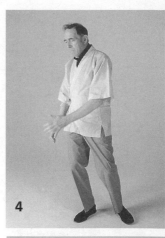

The left hand swings across the body to the right, the right foot taking the T'ai Chi step to the right, as the weight shifts (the waist turning), and the left hand continues in a circle. Meanwhile, the right hand begins a counter-circle to the left as the weight shifts in that direction and the waist turns. The circling arm passes by the opposing elbow—important—as the two arms circle in opposite directions. We do this movement 9 or 18 times.

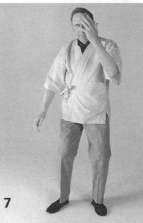 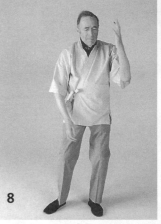

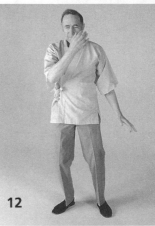

We close by bringing the feet together (right foot over to the left as in Figures 16-18) and coming to the rest position.

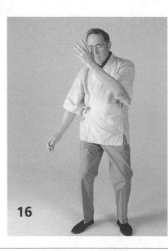

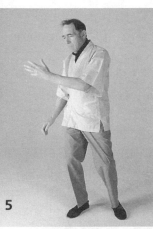

5

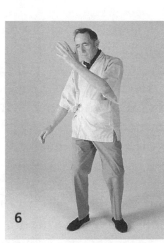

6

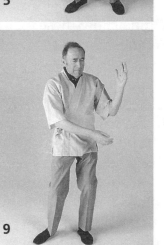

9

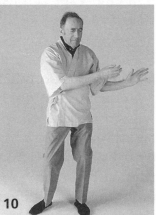

10

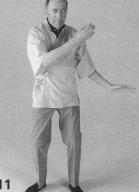

11

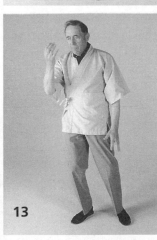

13

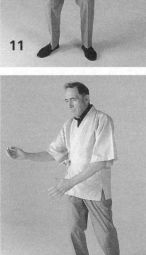

14

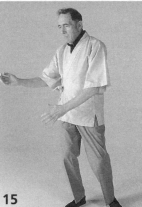

15

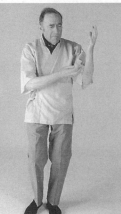

18

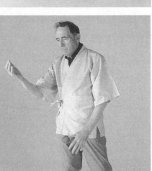

19

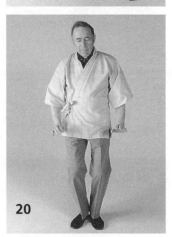

20

Six Healing Sounds

In ancient times there were two particularly strong influences in Chinese life. They were Confucianism and Taoism.

The teachings of Confucius were mostly humanistic in character. They had to do with correct social conduct, the art of governing, filial piety, observance of rites, and other similar considerations. As such, they have had a tremendous influence on Asian culture for 2,500 years, continuing until this day. Japan is largely a Confucian country, and owes much to the Sage's teaching.

Taoism, on the other hand, was generally mystic in nature. It is usually traced to the Sage Lao-Tzu, supposedly a contemporary of Confucius. The historicity of this wise man is sometimes suspect, but there is no doubt of the influence of the *Tao Te Ching* ascribed to Lao-Tzu and, according to legend, dashed off by him at the request of the frontier guard (himself an unusual man) who was the last to see Lao-Tzu before the latter left his kingdom and disappeared.

The *Tao Te Ching* has been translated at least 60 or 70 times into English, making it perhaps the most translated of all literary works, including the *Bible*.

The Taoists, who were close to nature and sought to flow with the current of the Supreme Ultimate (Tao, or T'ai Chi), cared not a fig for correctness. Lao-Tzu did not value education, morality, and other "virtues," which he said immediately created their opposites. In the world of oneness, such polarity did not exist. So, true Taoists, before the teachings degenerated into a second-rate religion, often spent time in the forests, or on mountaintops, in deep and solitary meditation. Many of the magnificent landscape scrolls of China show these shadowy Sages, looking rather small in the overwhelming scenes of waterfalls and rocky cliffs. Sometimes, in the background, we can just discern a hermit's hut.

Living this natural life in the wilderness, these wise men were, of course, exposed to hardships and disease. According to legend, they evolved a method of repeating certain sounds, synchronized with a motion resembling T'ai Chi Chih, in order to ward off illness or cure any indisposition. Each sound referred to a particular inner organ, and the idea was to concentrate on the appropriate organ while making the movement and slowly uttering the correct sound in a long drawn-out whisper.

These six sounds, with the organs they served and the Chinese character for them, are:

Ho (Heart)

Hu (Spleen)

Szu (Liver)

Hsu (Lungs)

Hsi (3 Heaters: below the navel
                 in the abdomen
                 between the eyes)

Chui (Kidneys)

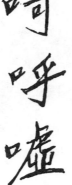

On pp. 84-87 will be found instructions for making the movement, on both left and right sides, and repeating the sounds. It is essential that these sounds be practised in good, pure air; next to an open window early in the morning, after finishing T'ai Chi Chih practice, is as good a time as any.

Six Healing Sounds

We step forward with the left foot, heel first, and push the left hand out vigorously while aspirating (breathing the sound, not speaking it aloud) the sound "Ho." We then pull back the left hand but leave the left leg extended, then push both hands out while aspirating "Hu" as we step forward again with the left foot, heel first. We then pull both hands back and bring the left leg back to the right leg, with a small space between the legs, and turn the hands, slightly above the waist on the right side of the body, so they face to the left. We then push the hands across the body while aspirating "Tzu" (Figures 1-9). Note the shift of weight as we push to the left, both palms facing to the left .

We then come back to the starting position and put the right foot forward, heel first, at the same time pushing the right hand out, simultaneously aspirating the sound "Shuh." We pull the right hand back and then push both hands out, aspirating "Shi" as we step forward again with the right foot, heel first. We pull the hands back and slightly to the left, turning the palms to the right, and push across the body as we aspirate "Chui," pronounced "Chwee" (Figures 10-18).

This is one set (Figures 1-18), and we repeat it twice more, so that, in all, we have done the entire sequence, ending with "Chui," 3 times.

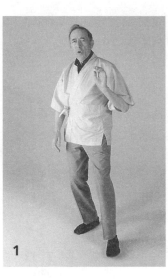

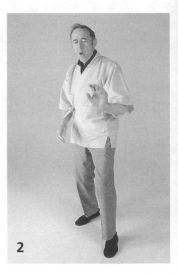

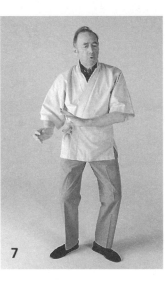

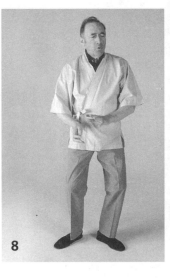

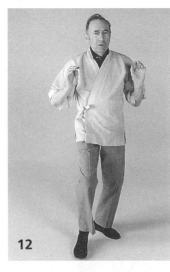

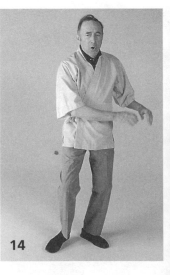

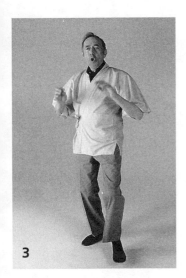

3

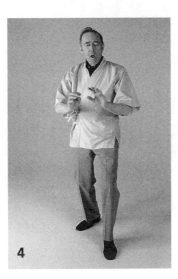

4

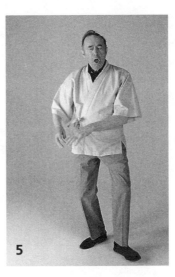

5

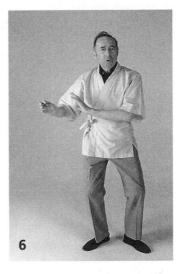

6

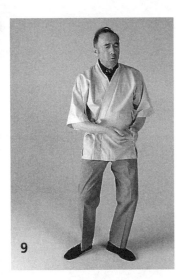

9

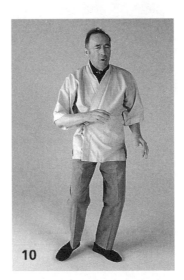

10

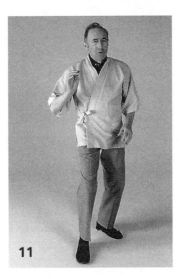

11

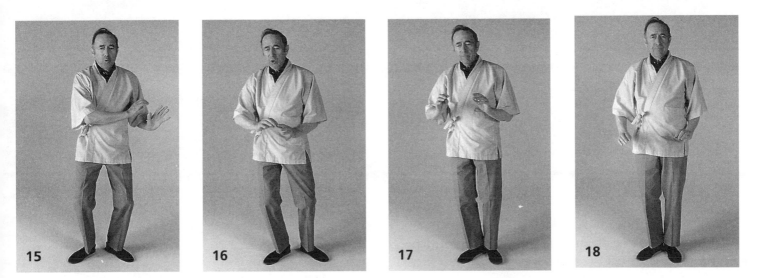

15

16

17

18

continued on pages 86-87

Six Healing Sounds (continued)

After the 3 sets just described, on the last sound "Chui," we turn the palms to the opposite side and push across the body, sounding "Chui"—then we turn back to the first side, push, and sound "Chui." In all, we push and sound "Chui" 5 times, back and forth, raising the heel and replacing it each time "Chui" is sounded (Figures 19-25), finishing on the right side. (The first "Chui" was on the right side, and so is the last.)

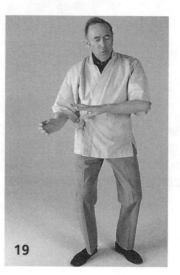 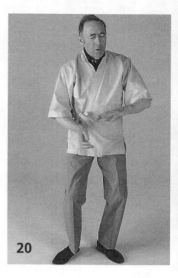

We then bring the hands to the sides in a graceful conclusion, palms facing downward and knees slightly bent (Figures 26-29).

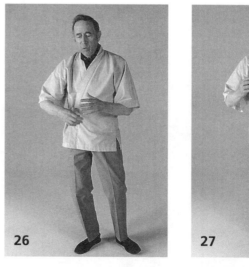

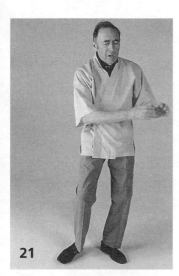

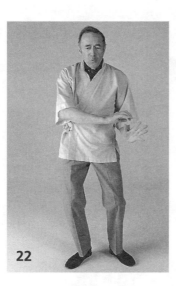

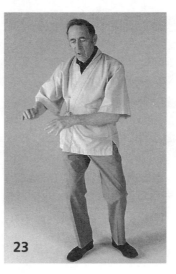

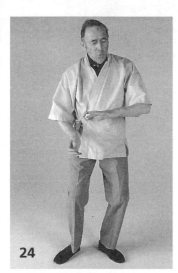

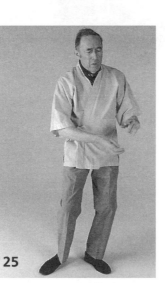

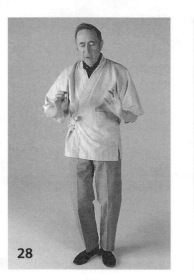

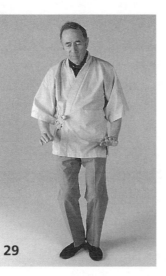

Cosmic Consciousness Pose

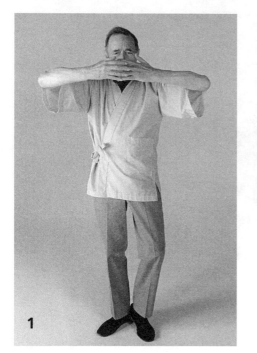

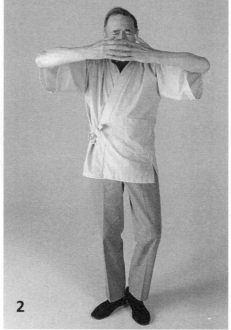

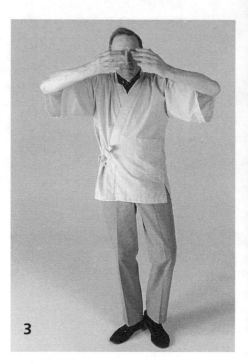

We usually take this pose for a short time, then come into the rest position. It is important to note that the left heel is raised and thrust into the side of the right ankle. Elbows should be level with the hands. Fingers are slightly spread apart.

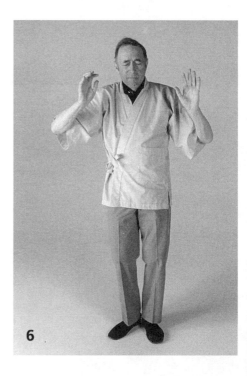

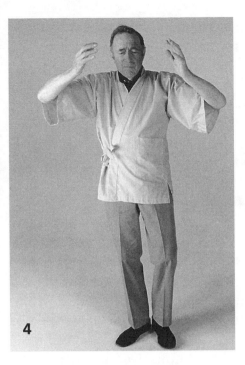

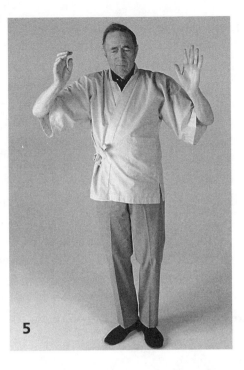

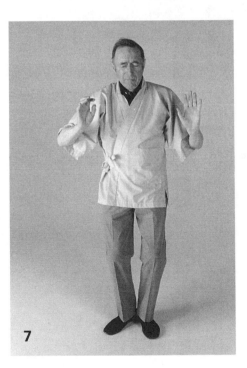

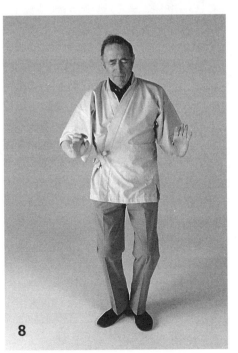

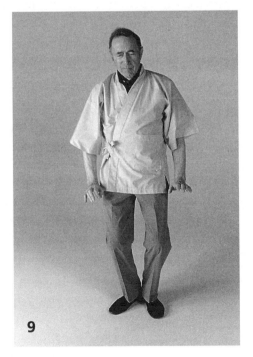

Notes On Movements Just Learned

Now you have learned the movements of T'ai Chi Chih. It is necessary to practise them regularly, not hard to do when you begin to realize how joyous such practice can be. Here are a few tips on what to remember as you do each movement:

Rocking Motion is a good way to loosen up and get the Chi to start flowing. Be sure the wrists are loose. Coming down, don't forget to land flat on the feet before lifting the toes; it is easier than rocking back on the heels.

In **Bird Flaps its Wings**, when the arms are out to the side the third time, do the wrist circles with the wrists, not the arms, and be sure a complete circle is made each time. We flip the wrists to the side quickly, but bring the arms and hands back together slowly. As the hands come together, the polarity of the palms facing each other is important, so do not rush bringing the hands together.

Around the Platter is done mostly with the wrists, starting at the chest. The hands are kept close together all through the movement. Be sure to settle down on a bent back leg as the weight shifts back, and straighten the back leg (not stiff and tense, however) as the weight moves forward to a bent front leg. Do not do stiff-legged T'ai Chi Chih! Observe the yinning and the yanging, the shifting of weight. Exaggerate it if necessary.

In *Around the Platter Variation*, be sure you carry a ball halfway around, then let it drop as the hands flatten out. Do not rush the backswing; slowly and evenly is the right way.

In **Bass Drum** we imagine a big drum at the chest, and we circle under the bottom and around over the top. Hands are about a foot apart and the movement is done mostly with the wrists.

In *Daughter on the Mountaintop* we start low because we are going high. (Actually, the two hands cross at about chin level.) The right hand is outside the left hand no matter which foot is stretched forward. After the two hands cross, do not point the fingers down but bring the cocked wrists downward with the fingers still pointing up until the very last moment.

In *Daughter in the Valley* we start high as we are going to go low. The hands swing in a half-circle, then start up with the palms facing each other, only a few inches apart. This slow rise of the hands as they come up is all-important because of the polarity caused by the palms facing each other. We are still shifting the weight forward until the hands begin to spread apart at the top of the arc. Do not begin to shift the weight backward before the top of the arc is reached.

Carry the Ball to the Side has several important points to remember. First of all, we have our hands cupped on the sides of the ball, and the ball is curved. As we move to the left and do an under-swing just below waist level, we slightly emphasize the right hand, but there is no emphasis as we swing up and over back to the right. Similarly, when we later step to the right, the left hand is slightly emphasized to balance the positive leg (bent with the weight on it). As we come up and over, moving the hands back to the left, there is no emphasis.

Push Pull is done with slight emphasis on the right hand as the left leg is forward. The emphasis is on the left hand when the right leg is forward. Remember that we push out and just slightly downward going forward, then turn our hands up and come up and over slightly as the weight shifts to the back leg. Do not push hard and keep your fingers pointing upward as you push forward. It is natural to breathe out as we push forward and breathe in as we pull back.

Pulling in the Energy is done with the palms facing upward, and, as we move the hands in a circle (as we did in "Around the Platter"), we visualize the energy coming into the fingertips from the most distant star. This is a simplification of imagining the five colored Pranas (Chi) coming in through the fingertips. In India it is felt that there are five major functions of the Intrinsic Energy, called Prana, and each one has a representative color. It is not necessary to know this; just use the energy from the stars.

Pulling Taffy seems to be one of the more difficult movements to learn, but it does not have to be; just remember that one hand, palm turned up, makes a horizontal pull below the top palm, turned down. The feet remain firmly on the ground; the heel is not raised. When the pull is finished, one hand is out, turned up to the sun, and the other is turned down near the back leg. The T'ai Chi sideways step is used, the leg snaking out to the side with the knee first slightly bent and the foot pointing to the side, not the front. Do not start with the two hands facing each other (a common mistake). The arms have crossed and then the hands pull past each other on a level movement. (It is not up and down like a dance movement.) And keep the feet on the ground!

The *first variation of Pulling Taffy* finds us moving to the front as we pull the palms past each other (and we are slightly pigeon-toed), then we bring the legs back in line and do basic "Pulling Taffy" to the side.

The *second variation of Pulling Taffy* is sometimes called "Wrist Circles," for obvious reasons. As we make two complete circles and one half-circle with our wrists (not the arms), we go up on our toes with each circle and then come down before starting the next circle. However, on the third—the half circle ending at the top of the loop—we stay flat on the feet and remain there, well-anchored, as we do the basic "Pulling Taffy" motion.

The *third Pulling Taffy variation* is often called "Perpetual Motion" as it is continuous. After we have pulled taffy to the left we sweep the right hand over (see photos on pp. 70-71) and it turns palm up to sweep to the right under the left hand, which has the palm down. Then we sweep the left hand across and prepare for the pull to the left. All this is done continuously with no resting point. After nine (or more) repetitions, we come to a graceful conclusion. If one were in a blizzard and wanted to develop warmth quickly, this movement would be a handy way to do it.

Working the Pulley is surprisingly easy, though it may look difficult. The hand that is pulled back, about waist level, moves slightly behind the body, then comes up just above the shoulder and pushes out in a swimming motion (see photos on pp. 70). When the left foot is forward be sure to turn, with the torso only, definitely to the left (not straight ahead), and when the right foot is forward turn the torso sharply to the right.

Light at the Top of the Head (and *Light at the Temple*) finds the feet held in one place. As the hands (really the wrists) swing out from the top of the head (or from the temple) three times, we rise on our toes and come back down as the hands come together above the head (or at the temples). Then we make a few circles, with the palms facing each other. When we eventually come down, in a wide circular fashion, the hands cross with the right hand underneath, and then circle back to bring them to the sides in the rest position.

Joyous Breath requires some pressure from the muscles, the only movement that does. We push vigorously down to the ground, breathing out deeply as we do so, and then pull up vigorously to the top of the chest as we breathe in *deeply*. Here we hold the breath for a few seconds, then start down again. This movement is so invigorating that some like to do it at the beginning of practice.

Passing Clouds is a very graceful movement. The hands move in circles, going in opposing directions, and each hand goes by the opposite elbow (it does not swing wildly) as it moves to the opposing side. We start with the left hand moving to the right, and we finish with the right hand moving to the left as we bring the right foot over to meet the left foot. In other words, we close on the left side.

The *Six Healing Sounds* are movements put to ancient Chinese Healing Sounds that Sages used when they lived in the forests. The sounds are not spoken aloud but are aspirated, that is, breathed, with barely audibly sound pushed out vigorously. In sweeping to one side or the other, both hands have the palms facing the direction to which the hands move.

The *Cosmic Consciousness Pose* is stationary, with the left heel off the ground, touching the right ankle. We look through slightly spread fingers and try not to have extraneous thoughts. This might be held 30 seconds or more, then the arms are lowered slowly to the sides.

PART THREE

Great Circle Meditation

If the reader would like to supplement his or her T'ai Chi Chih with a suitable meditation, to bring about an inner stillness after the movements he or she has been practising, this is an easy one to practise and should have great benefits. Carried to the extreme, it could be a way to Enlightenment. Somewhat similar methods were, euphemistically speaking, the "way to immortality" practised by ancient Taoists.

Instruction

Seat yourself in an upright chair, with the backbone held straight. (Those used to sitting in any cross-legged position, such as the full or half-lotus, should, of course, take that position.) After a moment or two of silence, with the eyes closed, adjust the breath so that it is flowing evenly, push the tongue against the palate (roof of the mouth), and open the nostrils wide.

Now we are going to take a current up the spine and down the front. To make it easier to feel, let's visualize it as a warm, golden, slightly moist light.

First, concentrate on the base of the spine (tailbone). Then, lift this warm, golden light slowly up the backbone. First, the small of the back, then the central part, the shoulder blades, the shoulders, the neck, and the base of the skull—thrilling each cell, as the current passes through, with the warm, golden feeling.

Next, the light reaches the top of the head, and we let it rest there for a few moments, the warm, golden feeling splashing down over the top of the skull and bathing us in its slightly moist, healing effulgence.

After holding the light at the top of the head for a short while, bring it slowly down the front—past the eyes, the nose, the mouth, the chin, and on to the neck; then, to the chest, the heart region, and the abdomen. Finally, it reaches the spot two inches below the navel (the T'an T'ien, or seat of heaven), where we let it stay for a few minutes, feeling the warm, golden current there, but making no effort to think about anything.

Now we are going to add two devices to make it easier to bring this warm, golden current up the spine.

1) As we move it up from the tailbone, we slowly inhale. By the time the current reaches the top of the head, our chest is expanded and holding its full capacity of air.

Hold the breath for a comfortable while. Let the light splatter down over the top of the head as we hold the breath, before starting down.

2) As we inhale and move the light up the spine, gradually raise the eyes from the spot below the navel, until they are pointed up toward the top of the head at the time the current reaches there and the breath is full. In other words, we use the eyes as a rope, or lever, to gradually lift the breath and the current, the three acting together. This should make it much easier to get the current to the top of the head (the "thousand-petaled lotus").

After holding the breath for a little while, as the eyes are pointed up and the current is at the top of the skull, we gradually begin to lower it down the front, at the same time slowly dropping our eyes (which are still closed). As the breath is gradually let out, we are careful not to do it in one long gasp, as this would call for an immediate reflex in-breath. Rather, we let it out in "sections," and, when the light is back down at the T'an T'ien, the eyes are pointing at the spot below the navel and the breath has come to rest. If it feels as if we are about to breathe in at once, simply force more air out and come to rest. This period of resting the current in the T'an T'ien, with the air out, is an important one. We are between breaths and, apparently, between thoughts. Make it a period of no mental activity as we rest in "ourselves." This is the full meditation, and it is suggested we make the full circle nine times, each time resting at the T'an T'ien below the navel.

We can make a larger circle by starting the breath at our feet. In this case, we "breathe" in through the soles of the feet (the "Hseuh" or "Bubbling Spring") and take the current up the inside of the two legs, before we bring it together at the T'an T'ien, and then through the opening between the legs and begin the trip up the spine.

In some esoteric practices, we "breathe" in through the sexual organ before going through the space between the legs and up the back.

If desired, when we are holding the light at the top of the head, with the breath held in, we can, mentally (eyes still closed and pointing up) repeat a mantra or affirmation. "Joy, joy, joyous joy" would be a good affirmation, or just the word "Joy." We can insert any positive state-ment we want at this point. It is an effective time to do so.

Practised regularly, this meditation can bring great benefit. It is up to the reader whether he or she wants to take the time to practise it once or twice a day after doing T'ai Chi Chih. Inci-dentally, at a boring lecture or gathering, or any time one can be silent for a few minutes (as on a train or plane), it is easy to close the eyes and do this beneficial meditation.

Epilogue

Let's talk about energy for a bit. While food is necessary, and we do derive some vitality from it, the true energy is the result of the Chi (Prana). If it were only a matter of food, an overweight person, or one who ate great quantities, would be the most energetic. But, is this the case? Overweight people are apt to be lethargic. Who wins the marathon race in the Olympic games, an overweight person? Hardly. It always seems to be a spare, underweight person described as "wiry."

It would be interesting to put some athletes on a program stimulating maximum Chi. The primary practice would be T'ai Chi Chih, and we would add the secret Nei Kung (practised while lying on the back), as well as certain breathing and meditative techniques. It is my guess that a track runner would then find he or she could surpass the best previous time for distance running and would reach a new plateau of performance. In such sports as basketball, an older player might find he or she tired less readily and was not as susceptible to the leg injuries that plague basketball players. A tennis player would, I believe, notice the difference in stamina in the fourth and fifth sets of long matches, and weight-lifters or shot-putters would find they could improve their best previous marks. I have never made these experiments, but am confident that an increase in the Chi, and better circulation of it, would readily accomplish these improvements. I have no doubts at all of the resulting improvement in physical fitness.

Many men find their sexual performance diminishing from the time of their mid-40s. Much of this, of course, is often psychological, but there is usually a definite physical slowdown in today's sedentary man after he reaches his 40s. However, T'ai Chi teachers in their 80s have been known to marry young women and have offspring. The Chinese respect T'ai Chi for its great aid to longevity. Just as important is the necessity of keeping vigor as one grows older. Chinese doctors for several thousand years have known that, when the yin and yang elements are out of balance, there is illness, and they have developed techniques, such as acupuncture (including massage and moxery) to right the imbalance.

So, when we lack energy, are chronically tired and lackadaisical, there is a good chance the Intrinsic Energy is not circulating.

In an excellent pamphlet, reprinted from *Chinese Culture* of March, 1969, the eminent teacher, Professor Huang Wen-Shan, says:

"We seem to realize that, in the universe, there is an ever-active, ever-creative life, and an inexhaustible source of energy-life and energy, which are made available to mankind when a fitting stage of development is achieved. It is particularly significant that it has a great reverence for life." So we discern a spiritual basis for this great Chi energy, which is not ours alone but belongs to the cosmos. (We manifest it individually when we do the necessary disciplines to develop and focus this great power.)

Professor Huang continues, "T'ai Chi (Supreme Ultimate) is originally circular in shape, and it is the combined entity of the yin and yang principles."

This circularity is the reason why, in all T'ai Chi disciplines, we move in a circular manner in order to activate this energy. A windmill follows the same principle.

"There is, behind the phenomenon of change, the Changeless Absolute, or Grand Ultimate (T'ai Chi)." From this we come to realize that, in working with this great force, we are doing more than mere exercise—we are pursuing a way to truth, or Enlightenment. Few realize that Enlightenment is experienced in the body, though this is what the Buddha and his successors have always taught and experience seems to prove.

"T'ai Chi is generated from 'Wu Chi,' or Ultimate Nothingness. It is the moving power of the dynamic and static states, and the source of the yin and yang principles. When they are in motion, they separate, and when they remain static, they combine. We can understand that…all its movements are in the patterns of the circular T'ai Chi diagram ☯ and they are expressed with curves emphasizing the principles of yang and yin, substantial and insubstantial motions, opening and closing mood, and dynamic and static state."

In the above statements, Professor Huang has quoted Chinese authorities of antiquity, and the principles apply equally well to T'ai Chi Ch'uan or T'ai Chi Chih.

Professor Huang refers to Wu Chi (Sunyata in Sanskrit), or Ultimate Nothingness. Whether we call this Nothingness, Void, God, or Buddha Nature, we are dealing with the same Great Reality. Just as Yoga attempts to retrace its steps so as to get back to the seed, or cause, in T'ai Chi practice we reintegrate by using our movements to take us back to the source. It is good if, after a period of movement, we do a short meditation, such as the "Cosmic Consciousness Pose" or the "Great Circle Meditation," in order to be quiet and centered while the great yin and yang forces, which we have separated and circulated with our movements, come together again. A very young and great Chinese metaphysician, Wang Pi (3rd century A.D.) has postulated, "Motion cannot control motion. That which controls the motion of the world is absolutely one."

The quiet meditation we enjoy immediately after T'ai Chi Chih practice, while our fingers, hands, and being are still vibrating, is a way to retrace our steps to this one that is the source. We do not have to be religious to do this. In this way we can make ourselves whole to go along with the great physical benefits we can derive from T'ai Chi Chih practice.

It is entirely possible to do the hand movements of T'ai Chi Chih while we are watching television or sitting in an upright chair—we simply place the appropriate leg in a slightly outstretched position to simulate the correct stance. A definite flow of Chi energy can be stimulated in this manner.

While walking down the street, I often find that, unconsciously, I am performing the T'ai Chi Chih movements with my hands—and with good results! Most frequently I seem to do the "Around the Platter Variation" movement or the difficult "Circles within Circles" movement (not included in this edition).

Do not be startled by the flow of energy, even if it is felt as a heat current at night and wakes you up. Go with this flow—rest in it and enjoy it. Sages have said it is the "Real," and they believed development of it led to long life. After continued practice, the reader should be able to estimate such benefits for him or herself.

Related Materials by Justin Stone

"T'ai Chi Chih/Joy thru Movement" (videotape)

Meditation for Healing/Particular Meditations for Particular Results (book)

"Justin Stone Speaks on T'ai Chi Chih" (audio tape)

"Spiritual Stories of the East,"– 2 volume set (audio tape)

Abandon Hope/The Way to Fulfillment (book)

Heightened Awareness/Toward a Higher Consciousness (book)

20th Century Psalms/Reflections on this Life (book)

Climb the Joyous Mountain/Living the Meditative Way (book)

Zen Meditation/A Broad View (book)

Spiritual Odyssey/Selected Writings 1985-1997 (book)

"Music for T'ai Chi Chih Practice & Restful Listening" (musical audio tape)

Contact publisher for complete catalog:
Good Karma Publishing, Inc.
P.O. Box 511
Fort Yates, ND 58538
701/854-7459
Toll-free: 1-888-540-7459

Please Note: Study of this photo-textbook does not constitute permission to teach T'ai Chi Chih. For information about accreditation courses, contact the publisher.